Reducing Cardiovascular Risk in People with Diabetes Mellitus

by Steven Levene

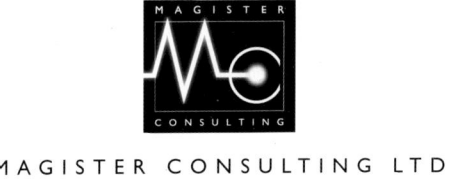

MAGISTER CONSULTING LTD

REDUCING CARDIOVASCULAR RISK
IN PEOPLE WITH DIABETES MELLITUS
by
STEVEN LEVENE MA MB BChir FRCGP

Published in the UK by
Magister Consulting Ltd
The Old Rectory, St Mary's Road
Stone, Dartford, Kent DA9 9AS

Copyright © 2006 Magister Consulting Ltd
Printed in the UK by Nuffield Press, Oxfordshire

ISBN 1 873839 67 7

This publication reflects the views and experience of the author and not necessarily those of
Magister Consulting Ltd.

Any product mentioned in the book should be used in accordance with the prescribing
information prepared by the manufacturer. Neither the author nor the publisher can accept
responsibility for any detrimental consequences arising from the information contained
herein. Dosages given are for guidance purposes only. No sanctions or endorsements are
made for any drug or compound at present under clinical investigation.

All rights reserved. No part of this publication may be reproduced, stored in a retrieval system
or transmitted in any form or by any means electronic, mechanical photocopying or
otherwise, without the prior permission of the copyright owner.

Contents

Foreword

Diabetics are certainly at greater risk compared with the normal population of developing cardiovascular problems in addition to their primary illness. Consequently, reduced longevity is a problem.

In the last couple of years there has been an increasingly powerful message to general practice that all diabetics should be on a statin in order to reduce the risk of cardiovascular incidents. More precise control of blood pressure in the diabetic is also required.

Many factors affect the development of diabetic complications and it is therefore important to have a structured approach to the problem in primary care where most management of diabetes takes place. There are a multitude of independent risk factors which need evaluation such as ethnicity, family history, obesity, lack of physical activity, excess alcohol and poor diet.

Add to this the effects of raised blood pressure and cholesterol, microalbuminuria and so on, the responsibility of the general practitioner and practice nurse in screening and using drug and non-drug interventions becomes very important. Because many of the risk factors are modifiable, interventions can produce very good results which improve quality of life outcomes.

It is, therefore, most desirable to have to hand a book of reference which can act as an aid to clinical practice, indicating the most appropriate and efficient assessment of diabetics in primary care in respect of their cardiovascular risk. The content of this book rightly reflects the cover title in that it most certainly is a practical guide for primary care and an immense asset to any practice library.

Dr Morris Pearlgood
General Practitioner, Eltham, London

About the author

L S Levene MA, MB, BChir, FRCGP
General Practitioner, Leicester, UK

Steven Levene trained at the University of Cambridge and St. Mary's Hospital, London. He has been a full-time general practice principal at a busy inner city training practice in Leicester since 1986. He has written several papers, mostly about diabetes, and a book on type 2 diabetes published in 2003. Apart from diabetes, his professional interests include pain management, training and research.

Acknowledgements

Many of the ideas in this book arose out of conversations over the years with numerous Leicester colleagues in both primary and secondary care. However, I am particularly grateful to two fellow GPs with a special interest in diabetes, Mike Drucquer and Azhar Farooqi, for their comments and advice, and to Sue Moriarty for her comments on some aspects of prescribing. The final responsibility for what follows is naturally mine.

During this project my family has had to endure a frequently "semi-detached" husband and father. In gratitude for their good-natured tolerance, I dedicate this book to them with love.

Preface

When I was invited by Magister Consulting to write a short book about diabetes, I quickly decided that the text should address two vitally important (but related) areas in the management of diabetes:
- the assessment of cardiovascular risk, and
- delaying the onset and progression of atheromatous disease.

The majority of patients with diabetes mellitus seen in a primary care setting have type 2 diabetes; many have (or are at risk of developing) serious complications affecting various organs or tissues, especially heart, kidneys, retina, feet and nerves. It is these complications that are responsible for the considerable morbidity and mortality associated with being diabetic.

The pathogenesis of diabetic complications starts with damage to large and small arteries. I hope that I can be forgiven for believing that diabetes mellitus is really a cardiovascular disease "masquerading" as a metabolic disorder.

Although the problems of diabetic patients can make considerable demands upon professionals' time and expertise, these patients stand to gain greatly from the delivery of high quality care - a fact that is recognised by the Quality Outcomes Framework (QOF) of the New GP Contract. Furthermore, much of the expertise acquired in diabetic care can also be used to help many other patients who do not have diabetes.

Practices are being bombarded constantly with guidance (occasionally contradictory) from various official or learned organisations. The frequent publication and dissemination of findings of different "landmark" studies, often with "interesting" acronyms such as UKPDS, LIFE, ASCOT, MRC/BHF, CARDS or ALLHAT, require that conscientious professionals need to review their practice on a regular basis. Sometimes, due to the amount of time required to prepare guidance, findings from the most recent studies cannot always be incorporated. As with any publication, even authoritative guidance risks becoming out of date over time.

Pharmaceutical companies regularly launch new drugs or adjust the marketing of existing drugs. These events are accompanied by intensive promotional campaigns designed to persuade prescribers of the value of these products in improving patient care, or even in helping practices to achieve one or more of their numerous clinical and/or managerial targets.

It is no wonder that many of us GPs suffer from information overload.

The busy non-specialist needs to know and then to analyse this steady stream of new information in order to decide how best to provide care for his patients. The gap between what is recommended and what can be achieved in an already stretched primary care service needs to be bridged, or at least minimised. The possession and deployment of relevant knowledge and skills should help practices to deliver higher quality care, and, hopefully, to reduce the effects of cardiovascular disease in people with diabetes - a particularly vulnerable group of patients.

The permanent prevention of cardiovascular disease is unrealistic in many patients with diabetes mellitus. What professionals should seek to do is to delay the onset and to minimise the effects of atheromatous disease.

Although a discussion of the available interventions to delay disease occupies the largest section of this book, it is important to recognise that the selection of the best treatment for an individual patient is helped by a better understanding of the concepts surrounding cardiovascular risk. Thus, there are separate chapters about the ways in which different factors contribute to this risk, the assessment of risk and its contributory factors, and how targets may be set for treatment. The relationship between these risk factors and cardiovascular disease can be both variable and complex.

Patients with type 1 diabetes are different from patients with type 2 diabetes in their age distribution and risk factor profiles. However, as stated above, most patients with diabetes have type 2, and most of the studies cited throughout the text involved patients with type 2 diabetes. Nevertheless, much of this evidence is also relevant to patients with type 1 diabetes, if interpreted with caution.

My aim throughout the book is to provide practical advice for the different members of the primary health care team who regularly look after patients with diabetes. I have tried to maintain a balanced perspective, but I hope that readers will accept (and possibly enjoy) my occasional digressions into related areas of particular interest to me.

The basis of our knowledge and skills in the fields of diabetes and cardiovascular disease is subject to constant change. The text is as up-to-date as possible at the time of going to press. I am optimistic that not many of the important concepts set out in this book will change radically in the near future. However, readers wishing to keep abreast of the latest information and guidance are advised to use as their starting point the resources suggested in Appendix 4.

Steven Levene
September 2005

Cardiovascular disease in patients with diabetes: its effects and risks

Setting the scene

As in many chronic diseases, diabetes mellitus poses a particular challenge to its sufferers and those involved in their care. Management of the disease should aim not only to eliminate or minimise current symptoms, but also to subvert a potentially disastrous natural history, i.e. improve future well-being. Thus, achieving and maintaining optimal glycaemic control needs to be complimented by other interventions to reduce the risks to a diabetic's future health.

Although diabetes mellitus is classified as a metabolic disease characterised by chronic hyperglycaemia, the pathogenesis of its complications and associated adverse events is frequently vascular, involving both the large blood vessels (the macro-vascular complications of coronary heart disease and stroke) and the small blood vessels (the micro-vascular complications of retinopathy, nephropathy and neuropathy). Unfortunately in the diabetic population, as compared to the general population, there is a considerably increased incidence of atheromatous disease. It is the devastating effects of atheromatous diseases which require a clear and aggressive approach aiming to prevent future mortality and morbidity.

Interventions to prevent future cardiovascular disease may require asymptomatic patients to undergo potentially unpleasant or even dangerous treatment. Successful prevention is more likely if both the patient and the professional understand the concept of risk and what factors contribute to increased risk. Furthermore, any preventative treatment needs to be compatible with the management of any currently existing disease.

What is risk?

It is essential to understand the concept of risk, used throughout this book, before looking more closely at the nature and effects of both contributory factors and interventions in cardiovascular disease.

One definition of the term risk, as understood by health care professionals, is the probability or expected frequency of harmful effects (due to a biological agent) occurring over a defined period of time. Choices need to be made about how to express risk. These include:

1. Quantified versus described risk

For optimal precision, risk should be quantified, i.e. a numerical value should be attached to it. However, in assigning a number to risk, the context and definitions need to be absolutely clear to allow correct interpretation of the figure. The drawbacks of using descriptions of risk, such as high, medium or low, are that these definitions may be unclear or may mean different things to different people. To enable clear understanding, a term should correlate the risk it describes to that of a commonly recognised event whose level of risk is understood: as with numbers, context and definitions need to be clear.

2. Absolute versus relative risk

The absolute risk of a particular event occurring over a specified period of time is usually expressed either as a percentage (a %) or a ratio (b incidences per a defined population size). Relative risk is usually expressed as a particular event being c % or d times more or less likely to occur in a defined population than in a compared population over a specified period of time. Where the absolute risks of two compared events or interventions are very low, small differences of risk may be relatively "large". For example, if a treatment reduces the risk of an adverse event occurring from 1% to 0.5%, then the absolute risk reduction is an unimpressive 0.5%, but the relative risk reduction is a staggering 50%. It is possible for the unwary to be misled by how numbers are used; a fact that does not escape copywriters in advertising.

The results of a risk-benefit analysis of an intervention are often presented now as "number needed to treat" (NNT). NNT is the reciprocal of absolute risk reduction. If a treatment reduces absolute risk by 1 in 10 or 10%, then the NNT of that treatment is 10. NNT is a better, much less misleading representation of a treatment's effectiveness than relative risk reduction.

Defining cardiovascular disease

Although the term vascular can refer to the whole of the circulatory system, it is sometimes used to refer to a part of the system. In order to be precise, the term vascular should be qualified in such circumstances to indicate which part of the circulation is being described.

In this book, vascular risk usually refers to the risk of developing macro-vascular or cardiovascular (CVD) disease, which is a combination of the risks for developing coronary heart disease (CHD), cerebrovascular disease and peripheral vascular disease (PVD).

In addition, patients with diabetes are at increased risk of developing micro-vascular disease, the mechanism for many serious diabetic complications (in eyes, kidneys and nerves) with potentially significant morbidity. The associated risk factors and modifying interventions discussed in subsequent chapters are also relevant to the pathogenesis and prevention of micro-vascular disease.

Why is cardiovascular disease important in patients with diabetes?

The rising prevalence of type 2 diabetes is associated with the increased presence of modifiable risk factors (discussed in the next chapter) that predict cardiovascular disease. When these risk factors are combined with a positive family history of CVD and/or the membership of certain ethnic groups, the relationship between diabetes and cardiovascular disease becomes even stronger and more lethal.

Cardiovascular disease is the cause of up to 60% of all deaths in patients with diabetes[1]. It is the commonest complication in Europeans with type 2 diabetes. Age-specific morbidity from CHD, cerebrovascular disease and peripheral vascular disease doubles in male patients and quadruples in female patients with type 2 diabetes, when compared to the general population[2]. However, patients with type 1 diabetes, especially younger ones, have the greater excess mortality from CVD over the long-term, although type 1 diabetics are usually younger than type 2 diabetics and may have different risk factor profiles.

Although the prevalence rate of CVD in patients with diabetes varies between populations, the presence of diabetes increases the prevalence of CVD in all populations. Among the aims of the management of diabetes, the reduction of cardiovascular risk surely has comparable importance to that of achieving and maintaining optimal glycaemic control.

The pathogenesis of diabetic cardiovascular disease

A variety of mechanisms contribute to the pathogenesis of cardiovascular disease in patients with diabetes. Although prolonged exposure of vascular tissues to raised blood glucose levels plays a significant role, other abnormalities are also very important: particularly those that contribute to insulin resistance (see Chapter 2). Some, such as adverse lipid profiles, precede the onset of type 2 diabetes, by which time atheromatous changes have already occurred. It is for this reason that the prevention (or if this fails, the early detection) of type 2 diabetes and its precursor, impaired glucose tolerance, needs to be incorporated into any delivery strategy for health care, particularly as the prevalence of diabetes continues to rise worldwide.

Vascular tissues exposed to high blood glucose levels develop several clinical and biochemical abnormalities, including changes to endothelial cells, vascular smooth muscle cells, glomeruli and mesangial cells, and cardiomyocytes.

Animal studies have suggested the following hypotheses for tissue damage resulting from chronic exposure to high glucose concentrations:

- Increased activity of the polyol pathway leads ultimately to depletion of myo-inositol and impairment of Na+-K+-ATPase activity, implicated in the pathogenesis of diabetic neuropathy.
- Accumulation of diaclyglycerol activates protein kinase C-ß (PKC) in endothelial cells, altering vascular permeability and increasing basement membrane synthesis. This may contribute to the development of new vessels in the retina (prolifrative retinopathy).
- Non-enzyme glycation is the attachment of glucose to the amino groups of proteins at a rate proportional to the mean serum glucose concentration, forming advanced glycosylation end products (AGEs). This is the basis for the glycated haemoglobin assay that measures medium-term glycaemic control. This long-term alteration of proteins appears to contribute to the development of atheroma in a number of ways; including protein cross-linking that produces oxidative damage and mononuclear cell chemotaxis that stimulates T-cells leading to increased macrophage uptake of AGE-LDL.
- Redox potential alterations: changes in free radicals and oxidation state.

It is possible that the precise pathogenesis of atheromatous change in patients with diabetes may vary not just between individuals, but also between sites and different calibre of arteries in the same individual. A better understanding of these mechanisms may help to identify potential therapeutic interventions, although a broad-based approach involving lifestyle modification and vigorous correction of raised blood pressure and dyslipidaemia must remain at the centre of reducing cardiovascular risk.

The costs of diabetes mellitus

It difficult to calculate the precise costs of diabetes mellitus to either the NHS or the economy, but we do know that these costs are rising. In 1997 one study estimated that diabetes care accounted for 9% of the annual NHS budget[3], greater than the proportion of the UK population with diabetes (3 to 5% of the population). As the prevalence of type

2 diabetes, with its associated morbidity and mortality, continues to increase, so will its costs. Much of this increased expenditure is consumed by diabetic complications, which are predominately vascular.

The Type 2 Diabetes: Accounting for a major Resource Demand in Society in the UK (T2ARDIS) project looked at the financial impact of type 2 diabetes and presented its results at Diabetes UK's Annual Professional Conference in March 2000[4].

T2ARDIS calculated that the average annual cost of treating each person with type 2 diabetes incurred direct costs to the country of £2152, comprising:
- £1738 (81%) to the NHS, the total annual cost being £2 billion, 4.7% of the total NHS expenditure, with hospitalisation consuming more than 40% of diabetes-related NHS expenditure.
- £285 (13%) borne by the private individual.
- £129 (6%) to the social services. Over 75% of social services costs for people with type 2 diabetes are associated with residential and nursing care.

T2ARDIS also showed that the presence of both micro-vascular and macro-vascular complications in an individual increased the average NHS costs in the calculation above five fold, personal expenditure three fold, and social services costs four fold. In 2005 these actual costs will be greater than in 2000, due to economic and healthcare inflation and to the rising prevalence of type 2 diabetes.

At Diabetes UK's Annual Professional Conference in April 2005, Professor Rhys Williams presented predictions that, by 2025, diabetes care worldwide could cost between $153 and 286 billions, accounting for 7.5 to 13.5% of total health care costs, a truly frightening prospect.

Any measures that reduce the medical effects of diabetes (by prevention, earlier detection or improved care to reduce complications) should also reduce the economic effects of diabetes.

The role of primary care in the management of diabetic cardiovascular disease

With the known prevalence of diabetes mellitus in the United Kingdom population being in the range of 3 to 5% and rising, and the increased morbidity of this population, it is clear that the management of diabetes mellitus and its complications is responsible for a significant proportion of each general practice's workload and budget. The sheer magnitude of the prevalence of diabetes and its associated morbidities means that the disease cannot be managed exclusively in secondary care. Primary care can and must play an important role.

The government recognised this by publishing a National Service Framework (NSF) for Diabetes in two parts, in 2001 and 2002, with the aim of setting out the standards and delivery of high quality care that need to be delivered to patients with diabetes throughout the National Health Service (NHS)[5,6]. The general practice contract was changed to reward the delivery of high quality care and the associated improved outcomes[7] starting in the financial year 2004/2005.

Both expert and central guidance have defined targets for care in diabetic CVD. Much of the responsibility for the delivery of this care will rest with hard-pressed non-specialist health professionals in primary care, rather than with secondary care. Great expertise is not required to assess and manage most adverse cardiovascular risk factors in an individual patient (although carrying out these activities in a population is a considerable undertaking in terms of time). GPs and practice nurses usually have a closer relationship with and better overall knowledge of individual patients. Patients have greater access to primary care, providing more and better opportunities to tackle CVD risk. Last, but not least, care delivery in the community is often more cost-effective than in a hospital setting, without loss of quality.

Although the challenge to reduce CVD in people with diabetes is colossal, primary care is well placed to "make a difference".

■ Key messages:

- Cardiovascular disease (CVD) is the cause of up to 60% of all deaths in diabetics.
- Reduction of cardiovascular risk is at the centre of diabetic management.
- The mechanisms by which prolonged exposure of vascular tissues to raised blood glucose causes damage are complex, not entirely understood and probably variable.
- The cost of diabetes mellitus and its complications to the nation is disproportionately greater than the numbers of people affected and looks set to rise in the future.
- Primary care plays a crucial role in managing diabetic cardiovascular disease.
- Government policies are now aiming to improve care for patients with diabetes.

What factors are associated with cardiovascular risk in patients with diabetes?

Overview

Chapter 1 introduced the concept of risk and considered the increased prevalence of cardiovascular disease in the diabetic population, compared to the general population. This chapter explains how different parameters, characteristics or factors contribute, both individually and collectively, to the overall cardiovascular risk in any single individual, particularly one with diabetes. Much research has been carried out or is in progress to study the absolute, relative and combined effect of different factors on an individual's global cardiovascular risk and what effect modifying them has on this risk. Not all factors affect cardiovascular risk equally, nor are all of them independent or susceptible to modification.

Risk factors can be divided into non-modifiable and modifiable (see Table 2.1). Obviously, only modifiable factors can respond to intervention. However, some non-

Table 2.1: *Cardiovascular risk factors and markers in patients with diabetes mellitus*

Non-modifiable risk factors	Modifiable risk factors
• Age	• Smoking status
• Gender	• Raised blood pressure
• Ethnic group	• Dyslipidaemia
• Family history	• Lack of physical activity
	• Poor diet
	• Obesity
	• Poor glycaemic control
	• Excess alcohol
	• Elevated fibrinogen
	• Cardiomyopathy
	• Raised inflammatory markers
	• Microalbuminuria
	• Hyperhomocysteinaemia

modifiable risk factors are needed to calculate global cardiovascular risk and, if present, can serve as a prompt to help identify those individuals in whom this risk should be assessed and "tackled", particularly in people normally considered to be at lower risk, such as those *without* diabetes.

Only the modifiable factors are discussed separately in the subsequent chapters on assessment and interventions. Of the above modifiable risk factors for cardiovascular disease (CVD), the following three have generally been regarded as the most important, both for their contribution to overall cardiovascular risk and for the resultant reduction of that risk when these factors are "corrected":
- Smoking
- Raised blood pressure
- Dyslipidaemia

The presence of evidence for the association of these three risk factors with developing a diabetes-related complication according to age, sex and type of diabetes is shown in Table 2.2.

Table 2.2: *Association of risk factors with having a diabetes-related complication according to age, sex and type of diabetes*[1]

Complication	Risk factor		
	Raised blood pressure	**Dyslipidaemia**	**Smoking**
CHD	T A G	T A G	T A G
Stroke	T A G		
PVD			
Nephropathy	T A G	T A G	T A G
Retinopathy	T A G	T A G	
Neuropathy	T1 A G	T1 A G	T A G

Key:
T = both types 1 and 2 diabetes in at least one study. T1 = known to be affected in type 1 diabetes.
A = known to be across all ages. G = known in both genders.

Currently, there is insufficient evidence to prove an association between diabetes-related complications and poor diet, obesity and lack of physical activity. Nevertheless, it may be reasonable to infer that, since all of these factors contribute significantly to global cardiovascular risk in the general population, any approach to reduce cardiovascular risk will usually need to address any adverse risk factors, and not just the "big three".

When considering both the assessment (discussed in the next chapter) and the correction (discussed in Chapter 5) of individual risk factors, readers need to remember that:

It *cannot* be assumed that the increase in cardiovascular risk attached to any particular factor will be matched by an equivalent reduction in risk if therapeutic interventions reduce or eliminate that factor. The relationship between cardiovascular morbidity and/or mortality and the reduction or elimination of individual risk factors is not always consistent.

Interdependence of individual risk factors

Although individual risk factors may have an independent effect upon the global cardiovascular risk, their overall effect upon cardiovascular risk is often more than additive, with different risk factors combining "at times… to become permissive for harm or create harm greater than that effected by simple addition[1]". In 1993 the MRFIT study demonstrated that the greater than additive adverse effect of a collection of risk factors is especially marked in diabetes, where the increase in risk attributed to any single or combination of risk factors is doubled when compared to a non-diabetic population[2]. There are still gaps in the evidence base. Matters become more complicated when evaluating the efficacy of various interventions.

However, there are recognised situations or scenarios where risk factors are clustered, e.g. metabolic syndrome (discussed later in this chapter). Furthermore, interventions that concentrate upon modifying a single risk factor may be much less effective in reducing cardiovascular risk than in having a multi-factorial approach (see Chapters 4 and 5).

Contribution of individual risk factors to cardiovascular risk

The contribution of each risk factor to cardiovascular risk in patients with diabetes is discussed below. To reiterate what was stated at the start of this chapter, not all factors contribute equally to cardiovascular risk, with some factors recognised as being particularly "dangerous" to patients with diabetes.

Age

Cardiovascular disease risk and the prevalence of type 2 diabetes both increase with age: this may be due, in a large part, to the greater prevalence of adverse cardiovascular risk factors with increasing age. The increased incidence of CVD with age is incremental rather than linear. It is more worrying (but not surprising) that the onset of CVD occurs at a younger average age in the diabetic population.

Gender

If the profile of other risk factors is otherwise similar, then healthy pre-menopausal females should be at less risk of developingCVD than their male contemporaries. However, in diabetic pre-menopausal females, this normally protective cardiovascular effect is lost[3]. There is evidence that the presence of a cardiovascular risk factor sometimes has a greater adverse effect upon women than upon men when diabetes is present.

A recent meta-analysis from Australia suggests that, whereas men with diabetes have a less than double the risk of dying from CHD compared to men without diabetes, women with diabetes are two and a half times more likely to die from CHD than women without diabetes[4]. Women also appear to be more susceptible to the adverse effects of both active and passive smoking upon cardiovascular risk.

Ethnic group

Due to complex and not entirely understood reasons, type 2 diabetes and CHD are commoner in certain ethnic groups, particularly in Indo- Asians, Afro-Caribbeans, Hispanic Americans, Native Americans, Fijians and many other non-white populations. This increased prevalence appears to be due to a combination of greater prevalence of other cardiovascular risk factors (which also produces greater insulin resistance – discussed later in this chapter), and an increased vulnerability to the effects of these risk factors. However, the presence of diabetes increases the prevalence of underlying CVD in *all* populations, irrespective of the level of original risk.

Positive family history

Patients with a family history of premature arteriosclerosis are at greater risk of developing CVD, particularly in a first degree relative, i.e. parent, sibling or child. This may be due largely to the increased prevalence (genetically mediated) of other adverse cardiovascular risk factors and an increased vulnerability to their effects. However, some families may also be exposed to one or more common adverse environmental components.

Smoking status

Half of all smokers die as a result of a smoking-related ailment. Smoking is a major aetiological factor for cardiovascular disease and peripheral vascular disease, as well as for lung cancer and respiratory conditions. There is a dose correlation between CHD risk and the number of cigarettes smoked daily.

Cigarette smoking increases cardiovascular risk by:
- Elevating low density lipoprotein (LDL) and lowering high density lipoprotein (HDL) cholesterol levels – see below
- Raising blood carbon monoxide (producing endothelial hypoxia)
- Promoting vasoconstriction of arteries already narrowed by arteriosclerosis
- Increasing platelet reactivity that may lead to platelet thrombus formation
- Increasing plasma fibrinogen concentration, resulting in greater blood viscosity.

Although the main benefits of smoking cessation are the reduction of all-cause mortality and the development of CHD, there is evidence now emerging that patients with diabetes may be able to reduce their risk of developing some diabetic complications, such as nephropathy and neuropathy by giving up smoking. Unfortunately, the proportion of patients with diabetes who smoke is the same as in the non-diabetic population[5].

Poor diet

The contribution of a "poor" diet to cardiovascular risk is its effect upon other cardiovascular risk factors: body fat (obesity), lipid profile, blood pressure, glycaemic control. It is not really an independent risk factor. Poor diet is not a straightforward measurable variable – such as serum lipids or blood pressure – and defies a clear simple definition. Modifying a poor diet is a potentially important means of improving other cardiovascular risk factors.

Lack of physical activity

A sedentary life style is associated with an increased risk of CHD, while regular exercise may be protective. Sedentary individuals are more likely to be obese and have adverse lipid profiles. In the United States, it has been estimated that the proportion of CHD deaths attributable to a sedentary lifestyle is in the region of 35%[6]. This estimate did not differentiate between non-diabetic and diabetic individuals.

Before getting carried away, readers need to remember that there is a lack of evidence demonstrating a direct relationship between physical activity and the development of the macrovascular and microvascular complications of diabetes. The arguments in favour of increased physical activity are based upon extrapolation from the effect of exercise on glycaemia. A recent report by the Chief Medical Officer distinguishes between the preventive effects (which appear to be strong) and the therapeutic effects of physical activity in people with type 2 diabetes[7].

Obesity

The World Health Organisation (WHO) defines obesity as "a disease state in which excess fat has accumulated to an extent that health may be adversely affected". Obesity with an abdominal distribution (also known as central obesity) rather than with gluteal fat accumulation is associated with metabolic syndrome and insulin resistance (see below) and a higher cardiovascular risk (particularly through dyslipidaemia), although it has not been demonstrated that obesity (as with lack of physical activity) itself is an independent cardiovascular risk factor in diabetes.

The WHO categorises body weight into: normal weight, overweight, obesity and severe obesity, using the body mass index (BMI), expressed as kg/m^2. However, the BMI is a measure of body *weight* and not of body fat or its distribution, whereas obesity indicates the presence of excessive fat, but not necessarily of excessive body weight: BMI and weight are not measures of the same thing. Some patients with diabetes have increased intra-abdominal fat but a normal range BMI.

Sadly, the prevalence of obesity is becoming an "epidemic", contributing to the relentlessly rising prevalence of metabolic syndrome and diabetes. In England 66% of men and 55% of women are classified as either overweight or obese[8].

Excess weight is almost always due to an imbalance between physical activity and dietary calorific intake: too little of the former in relation to too much of the latter. Any intervention to produce weight loss must, therefore, correct this imbalance (see Chapter 5).

Raised blood pressure

The importance of raised systolic blood pressure as a determinant of cardiovascular risk has been well documented in epidemiological surveys in many populations around the world[9,10].

The presence of both raised blood pressure and diabetes mellitus in the same individual is potentially a deadly combination. There is a rapidly increasing and strong body of evidence to demonstrate that raised arterial pressure is a significant, and potentially treatable, contributor to the development of major diabetic complications. Much of this evidence comes from several well-publicised trials involving patients with type 2 diabetes.

The effectiveness of the treatments studied in these trials is discussed in more detail in Chapter 5.

Unfortunately, hypertension is more prevalent in the type 2 diabetic population than in the non-diabetic population[11]. At a cellular level, diabetic individuals with raised blood pressure have increased sodium retention and increased pressor responsiveness, when compared to non-diabetic individuals with raised blood pressure[12]. In adults with diabetes, other atherogenic risk factors (Dyslipidaemia, elevated fibrinogen and left ventricular hypertrophy- discussed below) are also more likely to be present.

Dyslipidaemia

An abnormal lipid profile (also called dyslipidaemia) is a major independent risk factor in the development of CHD. Both cholesterol and triglycerides (TG) do not circulate freely in solution in plasma, but are bound to proteins and transported as macromolecular complexes known as lipoproteins; these are classified according to their density, ranging from very low density lipoproteins (VLDL) through low density lipoproteins (LDL), then intermediate density lipoproteins (IDL) to high density lipoproteins (HDL). However, TG is the major lipid group transported in the blood, with 70 to 150g entering and leaving plasma daily, compared with 1 to 2g of cholesterol. About 70% of the total cholesterol (TC) in plasma is carried in the LDL fraction and 25% is carried in the HDL fraction.

The combination of elevated levels of LDL with reduced levels of HDL predisposes an individual to the development of arteriosclerosis, regardless of whether or not diabetes is present. There is a direct and continuous association between total and LDL cholesterol levels in the serum and CVD risk, while serum HDL levels have an inverse correlation with CHD risk. The "hallmark" of obesity is the over-production by the liver of VLDL, which is then converted to LDL and is often associated with elevated levels of triglycerides. LDL levels may also be raised due to defective clearance, which has many causes, including reduced numbers or activity of LDL-receptors. Elevated levels of LDL and TG have a major adverse effect upon CHD risk. In contrast, HDL has several anti-atherogenic actions. When HDL-C is lower, the individual is more vulnerable to the dynamic features of atherogenesis (often mediated by raised LDL-C): these include cholesterol accumulation, inflammation, pro-thrombotic activity, matrix fragilisation and oxidative stress.

Cholesterol levels can be affected by both genetic (e.g. familial hyperlipoproteinaemias) and environmental factors, and by the presence of other conditions, such as hypothyroidism and obstructive liver disease. Individuals who migrate from a country with a lower prevalence of CVD to a country with a higher prevalence often alter their eating habits and other behaviours accordingly, resulting in a CVD risk closer to that of their new country's endogenous population.

The lipid profile is frequently "adverse" in patients with impaired glucose tolerance or type 2 diabetes: total cholesterol, LDL-C and triglycerides may be elevated, while HDL-C levels are often lower. Also, HDL-C is often "dysfunctional" or less active in patients with diabetes. As stated in the previous chapter, this abnormal profile often precedes the onset of pre-diabetes or diabetes by several years, so that atherogenesis may occur in advance of hyperglycaemia.

There is now strong evidence that improving the lipid profile (by both lowering LDL-C and TG, and elevating HDL-C) does reduce significantly the incidence of CHD mortality and morbidity (see Chapter 5).

Poor glycaemic control

The mechanisms of hyperglycaemia-induced vascular damage are discussed in the previous chapter. It has been suggested that there is a continuous relationship between the level of blood glucose and CVD[13].

The Diabetes Control and Complications Trial (DCCT) was carried out between 1983 and 1993 on 1,441 highly selected patients with type 1 diabetes. It demonstrated that "intensive" treatment improved glycaemic control and reduced retinopathy and microalbuminuria (a marker of cardiovascular disease), although a reduction in CVD was not demonstrated; mainly because the study looked at a young age group. However, serum cholesterol, an important risk factor, was lowered in the "intensively" treated group[14].

The UKPDS, looking at patients with type 2 diabetes, found that each 1% reduction in HbA1c is associated with a 21% reduction in the risk of a diabetes-related death, a 14% reduction for myocardial infarction and a 37% reduction in microvascular complications over ten years, with no lower threshold demonstrated[15].

Hyperinsulinaemia, which is present in many patients with type 2 diabetes, damages the vascular endothelium.

Excess alcohol

At least two studies found an inverse association between alcohol consumption and the risk of CHD mortality[16,17]. There is some evidence that moderate alcohol consumption may have some protective effect against stroke[18]. No data is available on alcohol consumption and the risk of developing peripheral vascular disease (PVD). Although there is no evidence to suggest that alcohol is a risk factor for the development of diabetic neuropathy, there are clinical grounds to recommend that alcohol is best avoided in patients with peripheral neuropathy.

Alcoholic cardiomyopathy may develop after ten years of heavy alcohol abuse. It is attributed to a direct toxic effect of alcohol on cardiac muscle. Alcohol abuse is also associated with thiamine deficiency, which can produce cardiomyopathy.

Elevated fibrinogen

Abnormalities of haemostasis are common in patients with diabetes[19]. Many patients with type 2 diabetes have impaired fibrinolytic activity associated with raised levels of plasminogen activator inhibitor-1 (PAI-1), which is the predominant naturally occurring inhibitor of tissue plasminogen activator (t-PA). The contribution of raised fibrinogen levels to CHD appears clear; their predictive value for cardiovascular risk may be comparable to that of serum cholesterol in both diabetic and non-diabetic populations[20,21]. However, as with some of the other risk factors, there is little evidence to support a direct relationship between elevated PAI-1 levels and diabetic vascular complications.

Non-CHD diabetic heart disease

Non-atherosclerotic heart disease occurs frequently in patients with diabetes and can co-exist with CHD, with adverse outcomes.

The presence of left ventricular hypertrophy (LVH) is associated with an increased risk of CVD and sudden death. LVH can be regarded as target organ damage to cardiac muscle usually due to inadequately controlled hypertension, although it can occur in diabetic patients, especially women, without hypertension. The presence or absence of LVH is used in some risk models based upon the Framingham data (see Chapter 3). However, LVH is not an independent risk factor that has a direct relationship with the development of diabetic vascular complications.

Diabetic cardiomyopathy results from worsening myocardial dysfunction, which often leads to accelerated heart failure[22]. Several factors are associated with the development of this cardiomyopathy. These include severe diffuse CHD, chronic hyperglycaemia, untreated hypertension, glycosylation of myocardial proteins and autonomic neuropathy. Pathological abnormalities in diabetic cardiomyopathy include myocardial enlargement, hypertrophy and fibrosis, and greater basement membrane thickening. The extent and nature of the resulting left ventricular dysfunction will depend upon which pathological changes have occurred.

Cardiac autonomic neuropathy (CAN) can evolve slowly in patients with diabetes. Cardiac parasympathetic nerve fibres are damaged earlier in the natural history than sympathetic fibres, resulting in a relative excess of sympathetic tone-tachycardia, reduced heart rate variability at rest, and a reduced response of heart rate and of blood pressure to exercise. Absent parasympathetic tone may produce increased coronary vasoconstriction, which may lead to ischaemia. Subsequent sympathetic nervous system dysfunction produces orthostatic hypotension. Autonomic dysfunction is responsible for the lack of pain perception for cardiac ischaemia, one reason why CAN is associated with sudden cardiac death in type 2 diabetics[23] and with increased mortality in type 1 diabetics[24].

Raised inflammatory markers

A recent paper in the *New England Journal of Medicine* has suggested that high levels of the inflammatory markers, C-reactive protein and interleukin-6, are associated with an increased risk of CHD in both sexes; but this effect is attenuated if diabetes and hypertension are present[25].

Microalbuminuria

Microalbuminuria is defined as the presence of low but abnormal levels of albumin (between 30mg/day and 300mg/day) in the urine. Although microalbuminuria, particularly if untreated (see Chapter 5 for details), has long been known to be a predictor of overt nephropathy and potentially end-stage renal disease (ESRD), it has also been shown to be a predictor of retinopathy, peripheral neuropathy, and hypertension, as well as an independent predictor of cardiovascular mortality and morbidity[26,27], particularly in patients with type 2 diabetes[28,29]. A UK study following 153 type 2 diabetic patients attending a hospital diabetic clinic showed an increased mortality, especially of cardiovascular death, in those with abnormal urinary albumin excretion[30].

Thus, it is reasonable is to regard microalbuminuria as having an additional predictive value for CVD mortality and morbidity in patients with diabetes, over and above that arising from diabetic nephropathy. However, there are considerably fewer management differences than previously between patients screening positive for microalbuminuria and patients screening negative. Interventions used in microalbuminuria, particularly drugs that block the renin-angiotensin aldosterone system (ACE inhibitors or ARB), are also commonly used now in diabetics who screen negative for microalbuminuria (see Chapter 5).

Hyperhomocysteinaemia

Raised levels of homocysteine (hyperhomocysteinaemia) are associated with coronary artery disease and nephropathy in cross-sectional studies among patients with both types of diabetes. There may be an association in these patients between hyperhomocysteinaemia and peripheral and carotid atherosclerotic disease and retinopathy, but not neuropathy. Hyperhomocysteinaemia is associated with an increase in all-cause mortality in patients with type 2 diabetes[1]. It is not yet possible to ascertain the precise cause and effect of these differences.

Metabolic syndrome

Insulin resistance is associated with a collection of abnormal risk factors (obesity, impaired glucose tolerance, hypertension and dyslipidaemia) and is now recognised as a major underlying contributor to increased CHD mortality.

Metabolic syndrome is a defined cluster of abnormal cardiovascular risk factors; its presence identifies individuals who are twice as likely to die from and three times as likely to have a CVD event, compared to people without the syndrome[31]. It also predicts the development of type 2 diabetes.

The two major previous definitions of metabolic syndrome were from:
- the WHO (including evidence of insulin resistance and measurement of fasting insulin), and
- the National Cholesterol Education Program (presence of three from the following clinical criteria: BP ≥ 130/85, HDL-C ≤ 1.04 mmol/l in men or ≤ 1.29 mmol/l in women, TG ≥ 1.69 mmol/l, fasting glucose ≥ 5.6 mmol/l or abdominal obesity)

In April 2005, the International Diabetes Foundation (IDF) proposed a new definition for metabolic syndrome that is appropriate for clinical use[32]:

In all cases: **central obesity**, defined as waist circumference in men equal to or greater than 94cm in Europids, Sub-Saharan Africans and Arabs, 90cm in South Asians and Chinese and 85cm in Japanese; and in women equal to or greater than 80cm, except in Japanese (90cm)

Plus any two of the following four factors:
- **Raised triglyceride level** (> 1.7mmol/l) or specific treatment for this lipid abnormality
- **Reduced HDL-C** (< 0.9mmol/l in males or < 1.1mmol/l in females) or specific treatment for this lipid abnormality
- **Raised blood pressure** (systolic ≥ 130mmHg or diastolic ≥ 80mmHg) or treatment of previously diagnosed hypertension)
- **Raised fasting plasma glucose** (≥ 5.6mmol/l- OGTT recommended to confirm diabetes) or previously diagnosed **type 2 diabetes**.

Epidemiological data about the metabolic syndrome is not entirely reliable due to its collection using different definitions, but it is clear that the prevalence varies amongst different ethnic groups, ranging from 22 to 39% of the adult population. It is commoner in an Indo-Asian population: a BMI greater than 23 kg/m² in Indo-Asians (as compared to 25 kg/m² in white Caucasians), is now thought to indicate increased CVD risk in this population[33] (subject to the occasional confusion of obesity with being overweight). Furthermore, these patients often have a low level of aerobic fitness, when compared to a control population.

Although no data is yet available from any large intervention trials in primary care for preventing or delaying diabetes or CVD in people with metabolic syndrome, there are strong reasons for taking an aggressive approach to managing metabolic syndrome, encompassing all relevant cardiovascular risk factors:

- Metabolic syndrome is clearly associated with a much greater risk of developing either CHD or type 2 diabetes or both.
- Its constituent adverse risk factors are also associated with increased cardiovascular mortality and morbidity, the result being often greater than additive.
- If these constituent factors are properly addressed, then mortality and morbidity are delayed or reduced significantly.
- Many of the interventions involve improving lifestyle, where successful change is known to be beneficial for more than CVD prevention.
- There is good evidence to support the effectiveness of many drugs in reducing blood pressure and regulating dyslipidaemia; better glycaemic control has also been shown to improve various outcomes.

Primary care possesses the skills, if not always sufficient resources, to screen for and manage metabolic syndrome. Interventions can be divided into primary prevention (moderate calorie restriction, moderate increase in physical activity and change in dietary composition) and secondary prevention (improve atherogenic dyslipidaemia, lower blood pressure, and correct hyperglycaemia or reduce insulin resistance). Further details of therapy are discussed in Chapter 5.

■ Key messages:

- Not all risk factors contribute equally to global cardiovascular risk.
- The most important cardiovascular risk factors are increasing age, non-white ethnicity, positive family history (not modifiable), and smoking status, raised blood pressure, and dyslipidaemia (modifiable).
- The adverse effect of individual risk factors upon cardiovascular risk is sometimes more than additive. Some risk factors may be interdependent. This has implications for both evaluation and interventions.
- Metabolic syndrome is an important risk factor for premature CHD in patients with type 2 diabetes. If present, it requires an aggressive correction of any adverse cardiovascular risk factors.

Assessment
– calculating global cardiovascular risk and evaluating modifiable risk factors in patients with diabetes

An overview

Having discussed in the previous chapter how different risk factors may contribute to the global cardiovascular risk, it is important now to consider how to quantify cardiovascular risk and measure the factors that contribute to this calculation. Every individual's profile of risk factors and his global risk are unique and will vary over time. Thus, an assessment to determine which risk factors are present, to measure them and to ascertain the global risk should normally be undertaken before planning and undertaking intervention. This process increases the probability that treatment will be effective and will address a patient's needs.

This chapter discusses not only the mechanics of evaluating cardiovascular risk and the factors which contribute to it, but also the interpretation of the data that may be elicited from such an evaluation. It follows that the presence or absence of CVD in the patient does not affect the mechanics of evaluating individual risk factors, but the presence of CVD will influence the interpretation of any data and should lead to a more aggressive approach to management.

Readers may find a recent review by Peter Winocour very useful when trying to grapple with the concepts surrounding the prediction of cardiovascular risk in patients with diabetes[1].

Screening for the presence of cardiovascular disease

Before proceeding to interpret any data derived from the evaluation of individual risk factors in the patient, the clinician should consider whether CVD is actually present.

The latest guidelines of the American Diabetes Association (ADA)[2] recommend screening with a diagnostic cardiac stress test if:

- Typical or atypical cardiac symptoms are present
- An abnormal resting 12 lead electrocardiogram (ECG) has been taken
- There is a previous history of peripheral or carotid occlusive disease
- Two or more major cardiovascular risk factors are present
- The patient is aged over 35 years with a previous sedentary lifestyle, but planning to undertake vigorous exercise.

This could be considered a counsel of perfection. Certainly, if there are clinical grounds to suspect the presence of CVD in any patient, whether or not with diabetes, the clinician's priority is to ensure that a prompt appropriate screening for disease is carried out. However, if only risk factors are present in the absence of any overt CVD and if the individual patient's circumstances so dictate, then the priority of clinician may be to reduce cardiovascular risk.

Differentiating between primary and secondary prevention of CVD is more interesting to epidemiologists than clinicians, and is often difficult in patients with diabetes. The diagnosis of CHD can be difficult, since the onset may be relatively "silent" in some patients with diabetes, especially those with microalbuminuria and/or autonomic neuropathy. Some strokes do not present with clear-cut neurological dysfunction or physical signs. The prognosis of individuals with silent CVD can be as poor as those with overt CVD. In any case, the incidence of CHD is higher in patients with type 2 diabetes.

Due to the considerations discussed above, some pragmatic clinicians make little distinction between primary and secondary prevention of CVD in patients with diabetes.

Risk models

The need to estimate cardiovascular risk more precisely

The prediction of cardiovascular risk has grown out of the need to identify a threshold beyond which interventions, in particular lipid modification, can be justified. An intuitive estimate of cardiovascular risk is unlikely to accurate. The combination of risk factors and their interdependent relationships makes it difficult to calculate the risk of a cardiovascular event occurring, either on an additive or on a piecemeal basis. Risk prediction tools have been developed to help treatment decisions, not just for dyslipidaemia, but also for hypertension.

The use of these tools requires the clinician and patient to understand the differences between absolute and relative risk (as discussed in Chapter 1). If the absolute risk is known, then the "absolute" benefit of altering a contributory risk factor can also be calculated for the individual patient (subject to the proviso stated in the previous chapter of the variable effect of intervention). By identifying those patients in whom absolute risk is greatest, clinicians (and managers) can be more confident that an appropriate absolute risk-lowering intervention will be both more clinically and more cost-effective. Such information is extremely important in any health care system where resources are finite and need to be targeted at those most likely to benefit from intervention.

However, two other important considerations besides absolute risk reduction need to be borne in mind before making any treatment decisions:

- Death by CVD can be delayed by effective interventions, but not entirely prevented; it remains the commonest cause of death in the western world.
- Other factors, such as increasing age, co-existing morbidities and the side effects of treatment, can have an adverse effect upon the quality of life in individuals without CVD. (Quality of life is sometimes measured in units called QALYs: quality adjusted life years). Preventing CVD in these individuals may be less important or relevant.

In these circumstances, making the right choices may be difficult for the busy caring clinician, with the added challenge of justifying potentially unpleasant or dangerous interventions to frequently perplexed patients.

The need for and role of risk prediction tools

Cardiovascular risk models have used data from the observation of a population cohort over a period of time, based upon the recording of risk factors and of CVD events. The usefulness of a risk model depends upon whether the calculation takes account of all important contributory risk factors and whether the important demographics of the individual being assessed are adequately represented in the population used in the model.

The need to treat "severe" hypertension in cerebrovascular and coronary heart disease is certain; reference to a cardiovascular risk prediction tool is unnecessary. However, it is prudent that a decision to treat "moderate" or borderline hypertension should follow an assessment of CHD risk, using a prediction tool applied in the same way as to dyslipidaemia.

Winocour has pointed out that "the outcome data for treating serum lipids and hypertension would suggest that CHD (not all CVD) outcome is more likely to be improved by hypolipidaemic as opposed to hypotensive therapy[1]." For stroke reduction in patients aged less than 55, the benefits of treating hypertension are likely to be affected by an associated dyslipidaemia. In contrast, the absolute risk of developing cerebrovascular disease is high in the elderly: blood pressure control is likely to be required independently of blood lipid and/or glucose levels.

Risk prediction tables have been used in the UK since the mid 1990s. At that time the high cost of lipid-lowering was a political issue and the Department of Health recommended a threshold of annual risk for a CHD event of 3% (eventually to be lowered to 1.5%, resources permitting), above which the prescription of expensive drugs could be justified.

Risk models based upon Framingham data

Many risk models have derived their data from the Framingham Heart Study, which was undertaken in 1948 and 1971 by the National Heart Institute in the United States and which followed up a cohort of just over 5,000 individuals without manifest cardiovascular disease in a town in Massachusetts.

Models that use the Framingham database include the Modified Sheffield Table, the updated New Zealand Calculator, the Canadian Graph, the Revised Joint British Societies Graph and Calculator, and the Joint European Guideline Chart. These models predict risk for CVD, CHD or stroke, either over a period of 5 or 10 years or annualised. The age limits for these models range from 26 to 40 years at the lower end to 70 to 74 years at the upper end. The factors included in the calculations are age, gender, smoking status, blood pressure (some include only systolic blood pressure), lipid profile (total cholesterol and high-density lipoprotein), the presence or absence of diabetes, and the presence or absence of left ventricular hypertrophy. The formats in which the results of these calculations are presented include tables, charts and computer programmes by several authors.

Interestingly, comparison of the results from various Framingham-derived models with the original Framingham algorithm shows considerable variation, with none of the models showing uniformly high (greater than 90%) sensitivity and specificity at both low and high thresholds of risk. The Modified Sheffield Table and the Revised Joint British Societies Graph and Calculator came out best in this comparison[3].

As a tool to predict cardiovascular risk in the current UK population, the Framingham database with its various derived models has several weaknesses:

1. The estimates apply only to those without known heart disease.
2. Some of the models predict heart disease only and not stroke.

3. The data was captured over 30 years ago when many of the treatments currently used were not yet available.
4. The Framingham cohort was predominately white, with few blacks and no South Asians.
5. There were only 337 people with diabetes in the Framingham database.
6. The derived models give risk over a fixed time span of 5 or 10 years, but not lifetime or longer term risk. Thus, they may have less value in predicting risk in a younger age group.
7. Family history, an important predictor of risk, is not included in the calculation.
8. Data in some tables do not differentiate clearly baseline blood pressure from levels achieved on treatment.
9. Triglyceride data is not incorporated into the tables.

Therefore, any calculation derived from a model derived from Framingham data must be applied with caution.

Other cohorts

In addition to the Framingham cohort, several other geographical and time-based cohorts have been used to generate risk models. Among the most interesting ones are:

- The German PROCAM study was an observational study in the 1970s run along similar lines to Framingham[4]. However, PROCAM recruited only men and included only 400 diabetics.
- Menotti et al[5] looking at a smaller rural Italian cohort, found much lower levels of absolute risk than Framingham, now referred to as the "Mediterranean effect".
- Pocock et al[6] combined the findings of 8 randomised controlled trials (RCTs) in Europe and North America to assess the risk of CVD death (not a non-fatal event- this is a disadvantage) in hypertensive individuals. Unlike the Framingham model, this model could incorporate existing cardiovascular disease markers into its estimate.
- The Cardiovascular Disease Life Expectancy Model[7] is based upon the results of 9 RCTs, estimating years of life saved by modelling changes in the progression of coronary and cerebrovascular disease over an average patient's lifetime. This has an advantage over other models of removing the 5 or 10 year duration, but this model is currently unavailable in an accessible form for use during a consultation.
- The SCORE Model estimates the 10 year risk of fatal cardiovascular disease in high and low risk populations, based upon cohort data from 12 European countries[8]. SCORE has the drawbacks of not providing separate scores for patients with diabetes and of not recognising non-fatal events as end points.

The drawbacks of existing risk models

Thus, each of the other risk models is also flawed. Some of the drawbacks are the same as in the Framingham model. Table 3.1 summarises the problems that can arise from using cardiovascular risk prediction tools.

Table 3.1: *Potential drawbacks of cardiovascular risk prediction tools*

Applicable to both diabetic and non-diabetic populations

- The use of shorter fixed time spans, as opposed to long-term or lifetime
- Annualised risk does not reflect the incremental increased incidence of CVD with age
- Failure to include all the relevant risk factors contributing to cardiovascular risk
- The lack of valid data for certain ethnic groups
- Failure to take into consideration the confounding effect of modern treatments
- Different risk engines will give different risk predictions with the same data.

Applicable to a diabetic population

- Under-representation of people with diabetes in the study populations, leading to a smaller database upon which to base calculations of risk.
- While risk models regard diabetes as a categorical variable, they ignore the level of glycaemia, which is probably an important predictor of CVD and CHD in patients with type 2 diabetes[9]
- Failure to include important markers or factors associated with increased cardiovascular risk in patients with diabetes, such as microalbuminuria and raised serum triglycerides

In the risk engines listed above, as well as the UKPDS engine discussed below, risk is "annualised", i.e. expressed as a percentage likelihood of an adverse event occurring in one or a defined number of years. However, this creates an artificial and possibly erroneous impression of cardiovascular risk.

The rate at which the incidence of CVD increases with age is probably incremental rather than linear. This creates the practical difficulty of where exactly to place an individual within the timescale of a risk engine, particularly as the duration of exposure to a risk marker has to be assumed and may be inaccurate, particularly in diabetes. Although risk is commonly presented over a 5 or 10 year period, it does not necessarily pinpoint that point in time which represents accurately an individual's risk. In the Framingham calculation, there is little difference in the annualised age-corrected risk between years 1 and 10.

Thus, bearing in mind that people with diabetes tend to be under-represented in many of the databases used for risk calculation, annualisation of risk may not be an accurate way of predicting cardiovascular events in patients with diabetes.

The UKPDS database

In an attempt to produce a prediction tool better suited to a diabetic population, the UKPDS (United Kingdom Prospective Diabetes Study) database was used to produce a diabetes-specific risk engine[10] (also available online: http://www.dtu.ox.ac.uk) to predict annual CHD risk (defined as fatal or non-fatal MI or sudden death). The calculation incorporates HbA1c, systolic blood pressure, TC: HDL-C ratio, age, sex, ethnic group, smoking status and time elapsed since diabetes was diagnosed. The engine can also report the different levels of risk for CHD, PVD and cerebrovascular disease. Another advantage of the UKPDS database over other databases is that it is based upon an interventional study.

However, the UKPDS database and risk engine do have the following drawbacks:
- The risk engine has only been validated in a type 2 diabetes population
- The calculation does not include microalbuminuria, family history, triglycerides or ECG findings
- The effects of aspirin, other anti-platelet agents and smoking cessation were not stated.

The UKPDS risk engine is a more "refined" tool to predict cardiovascular risk in diabetics without evident CVD. However, despite "imperfections", using one of the models derived from the Framingham data is currently the best way to estimate cardiovascular risk in untreated Northern European patients, provided that caution is used when applying the actual results. To produce a more accurate figure in patients of South Asian ethnicity or with a first degree relative who suffered a premature CVD event, clinicians should consider multiplying the result of a Framingham calculation by 1.5 (if both factors are present, the result could be doubled). Although crude, this manoeuvre may partly counteract two drawbacks of a Framingham-derived model.

Ultimately, such arguments may be less relevant when estimating cardiovascular risk in patients with diabetes, since all of these individuals should be regarded as being at greater risk of developing cardiovascular disease than members of the non-diabetic population and require more aggressive management of all relevant risk factors, irrespective of baseline and initial risk calculation.

Smoking status

This can be determined by asking the patient. If the patient is a current smoker, it is also useful to ascertain the patient's attitude to smoking cessation, previous attempts to stop, and what barriers are present to prevent the patient from stopping.

Diet

As in smoking and other risk factors that result mainly from the patient's life style, the professional should seek to gather information not just about current behaviour, but about willingness and barriers to change. The assessment may gather information from questioning both the patient and other members of the household, and from asking the patient to compile a food diary.

The components of a nutritional assessment might include:
- **Meal pattern:** the usual pattern of meals and snacks throughout the day. It is also important to elicit the extent to which this varies from day to day, between weekdays and weekends, and the influence of factors such as working patterns, travel and school (where applicable).
- **Food choices:** the types of and typical quantities consumed of foods that make up these meals and snacks.
- **Overall dietary balance:** How closely does the current diet correspond to "Balance of Good Health" guidelines*, particularly how much fruit and vegetables are consumed?
- **Nutritional adequacy:** Is there a dietary surplus or deficiency?
- **Alcohol consumption:** Does this exceed the safe limits? (see below)
- **Beliefs or misconceptions relating to diabetes and diet:** These might include sugar is forbidden or diabetic food products are essential.

At the end of a dietetic assessment, the professional should have sufficient information to help the patient to set achievable dietary goals.

---

*The Balance of Good Health is a nationally agreed model for dietary advice.
The model divides foods into five groups:
- Fruit and vegetables – recommending that 5 portions (400g) are eaten daily
- Bread, other cereals and potatoes – recommending 5 portions per day and aiming for high fibre kinds
- Milk and dairy foods – choosing lower fat alternatives
- Meat, fish and alternatives – aiming for smaller portions (a maximum of 2 portions per day) and lower fat alternatives
- Fatty and sugary foods – aiming to reduce quantities

Obesity

To calculate body mass index (BMI), the height and weight of the patient need to be measured. The calculation is done automatically when the data is entered correctly onto a software system such as EMIS. The calculation to be done is:

BMI = weight (in kilogrammes) divided by the square of height (in metres).

However, as discussed above, calculating BMI is not necessarily an accurate measure of body fat, in particular intra-abdominal fat. Furthermore, the BMI ranges are characteristic of a white population. Measuring skin fold thickness can under-estimate body fat in individuals with central obesity rather than with gluteal fat accumulation. Although calculation of the waist-hip ratio (WHR) has been used, it may under-estimate intra-abdominal obesity if gluteal obesity is also present. Calculation of the waist circumference (measured half way between the lowest point of the rib cage and the iliac crest) is a suitable easily measurable criterion for long-term follow-up[11]. Furthermore, as increased waist circumference has just been proposed as an essential criterion for the diagnosis of metabolic syndrome (see the end of Chapter 2), it could be argued that this measurement is more important than BMI for evaluating cardiovascular risk.

In 2003 Diabetes UK produced a stratification of co-morbidity risk, correlated with BMI and waist circumference in adults, summarised in Table 3.2. In a Caucasian population,

Table 3.2: *Co-morbidity risks associated with different levels of BMI and waist circumference (from Diabetes UK)[12]*

	Caucasian Waist circumference (cm)		Asian-Pacific Waist circumference (cm)	
Male	<102	≥102	<90	≥90
Female	<88	≥88	<80	≥80
Risk of co-morbidity	**BMI**	**BMI**	**BMI**	**BMI**
Low (but ↑other risks)	<18.5		<18.5	
Average	18.5 – 24.9	<18.5	18.5 – 22.9	<18.5
Increased	25.0 – 29.9	18.5 – 24.9	23.0 – 24.9	18.5 – 22.9
Moderate	30.0 – 34.9	25.0 – 29.9	25.0 – 29.9	23.0 – 24.9
Severe	35.0 – 39.9	30.0 – 34.9	30.0 – 34.9	25.0 – 29.9
Very Severe	≥40.0	≥35.0	≥35.0	≥30.0

a waist circumference ≥102 cm in men and ≥88 cm in women predicts an increased risk of disease associated with obesity; while in an Asian-Pacific population, the threshold is ≥90 cm in men and ≥80 cm in women.

Blood pressure

Due to pressures of time and less than ideal ergonomics, many health professionals (the author included!) do not invariably measure a patient's blood pressure correctly. Detailed authoritative guidance on how it should be done is given in Table 3.3, again a counsel of perfection.

A variety of automated sphygmomanometers are now available for professional and self-use. Before purchasing any model, the buyer is advised to enquire whether the device has passed independent validation using the protocols of the British Hypertension Society (BHS) and the Association for the Advancement of Medical Instrumentation Standard (AAMI)[13]. Further useful advice may be available from the local hospital's medical physics department. Mercury sphygmomanometers are *still* legal and they can be as accurate (when set up properly) as the best automated machine. Many aneroid sphygmomanometers lose accuracy when jolted.

Further independent evaluation of the available blood pressure measuring devices is being undertaken and may be published at some point in the future.

Serum lipids

Serum lipid estimation is best done after an overnight fast, because chylomicrons from the last meal can affect triglyceride levels. The practice should request that the local chemical pathology laboratory provides total cholesterol, lipoprotein fractions, and triglyceride levels in its report. Most laboratories will give LDL-cholesterol and HDL-cholesterol values.

Table 3.3: *Guidelines for Blood Pressure Measurement*[3,14,15]

Measure sitting blood pressure routinely: standing blood pressure should be recorded at least once at the initial estimation in elderly or diabetic patients

- Standardise the environment as much as possible:
  - remove tight clothing
  - relaxed temperate setting, with the patient seated
  - arm for measurement to be positioned out-stretched, in line with mid-sternum, and supported at heart level
  - avoid talking during measurement
  - use a properly maintained, calibrated, and validated device.
- Correctly wrap a cuff containing an appropriately sized bladder around the upper arm and connect to a manometer. Cuffs should be marked to indicate the range of permissible arm circumferences; these marks should be easily seen when the cuff is being applied to an arm.
- Palpate the brachial pulse in the antecubital fossa of that arm.
- Rapidly inflate the cuff to 20 mmHg above the point where the brachial pulse disappears.
- Deflate the cuff and note the pressure at which the pulse re-appears: the approximate systolic pressure.
- Re-inflate the cuff to 20 mmHg above the point at which the brachial pulse disappears.
- Using one hand, place the stethoscope over the brachial artery ensuring complete skin contact with no clothing in between.
- Slowly deflate the cuff at 2–3 mmHg per second listening for Korotkoff sounds. Read blood pressure to the nearest 2 mm Hg.
  - Phase I: The first appearance of faint repetitive clear tapping sounds gradually increasing in intensity and lasting for at least two consecutive beats: note the **systolic pressure**.
  - Phase II: A brief period may follow when the sounds soften or 'swish'.
  - Auscultatory gap: In some patients, the sounds may disappear altogether.
  - Phase III: The return of sharper sounds becoming crisper for a short time.
  - Phase IV: The distinct, abrupt muffling of sounds, becoming soft and blowing in quality.
  - Phase V: The point at which all sounds disappear completely: note the **diastolic pressure**.
- When the sounds have disappeared, quickly deflate the cuff completely, if repeating the measurement.
- When possible, take readings at the beginning and end of consultations. Take the mean of at least two readings. More recordings are needed if marked differences between initial measurements are found.
- Do not treat on the basis of an isolated reading.

Glycaemic control

Glycaemic control can be assessed in three complementary ways:
- Glycosylated haemoglobin
- Patient self-monitoring of either blood or urinary glucose
- Patient symptoms.

Glycosylated haemoglobin

Glycosylated haemoglobin, or HbA1c, is a useful measure of glycaemic control. HbA1c is formed by the non-enzyme glycation of part of the ß-chain cell haemoglobin. HbA1c levels reflect the *mean* plasma glucose over the preceding 6 to 8 weeks. The relationship between HbA1c and mean plasma glucose levels is shown in Table 3.4. Measurement of HbA1c requires expensive equipment and stringent quality control: it is best done in a hospital laboratory.

Table 3.4: Correlation between HbA1c level and mean plasma glucose levels[16]

HbA1c (%)	Mean plasma glucose level (mmol/l)
6	7.5
7	9.5
8	11.5
9	13.5
10	15.5
11	17.5
12	19.5

Patient self-monitoring of either blood or urinary glucose

Testing urine for the presence of glucose using test strips, such as Diabur-Test 5000, is non-invasive, inexpensive and may be preferred by patients who dislike blood testing (although there is some recent evidence that patients with type 2 diabetes can have negative perceptions about urine testing[17]).

However, urine glucose testing has two main limitations:
1. The quantity of glucose, if any, in a sample of recently formed urine is more indicative of the mean blood glucose levels over the period of time when the urine was formed than of the blood glucose level at a given moment. Urine levels of glucose do not reflect any sudden fluctuation in blood glucose levels and are, thus, inexact.
2. In some type 2 patients, the renal threshold for glycosuria is abnormally high or low. Thus, it is possible for no glycosuria to be present with a moderately raised blood glucose level, or for glycosuria to be present with a normal blood glucose level.

Despite these "disadvantages", if diabetic control is adequate with urine testing (i.e. good HbA1c, infrequent hypoglycaemia), then blood testing may not be necessary in patients with type 2 diabetes on diet alone or oral medication.

Blood glucose testing is recommended for diabetic patients treated with insulin (both types 1 and 2), and may be desirable in patients on diet alone or oral medication, who require accurate estimations of their blood glucose.

Blood glucose testing is more expensive than urine testing. Many varieties of finger-pricking lancets, blood glucose machines and test strips are now available, but only the lancets and strips can be prescribed on an FP10 prescription form. Each different make of blood glucose machine has its own unique test strips. The current issue of the Monthly Index of Medical Specialities (MIMS) lists each make of test strip and the machine(s) with which it is compatible. There have been significant technical advances in machines, with sensors allowing the blood drop to be analysed outside the machine. It is vital to remember that plasma glucose values are 11% higher than whole blood values. Machines will be calibrated to one of these.

Although blood glucose machines are not available on prescription, many are inexpensive, often costing less than £20. If the GP writes a letter confirming the diagnosis of diabetes, then the patient is exempt from paying Value Added Tax (VAT) at purchase, provided that the machine is intended for that patient's personal use.

A rigorous evaluation of the different blood glucose meters and lancing devices now available on the UK market was published in April 2005 by the Department of Health's

Medicines and Healthcare products Regulatory Agency (details can be downloaded from its website, www.mhra.gov.uk). This source of useful and clearly set out information should help any individual to select the most suitable device for his needs.

Health education is an essential component of self-monitoring. The correct use of a correctly calibrated blood glucose measuring machine and the appropriate interpretation of results are essential. Lancets need to be disposed of safely; preferably using either a needle clip or a sharps bin (both can be prescribed).

Most official guidance and Diabetes UK do favour regular home blood glucose monitoring, even in type 2 diabetics, but there is not yet a clear consensus on how frequently to test. The latest ADA guidelines recommend 2 to 3 times daily in patients with type 1 diabetes, but possibly more often in patients with type 2 diabetes on insulin[2]. However, a recent editorial in the *British Medical Journal* challenged the conventional advice given about frequency of testing; it suggested that regular monitoring is necessary only in certain situations and that properly conducted large scale studies need to be done to determine whether more frequent testing will improve glycaemic control[18].

Patient symptoms

Patient well-being is a much less precise and a potentially misleading method of assessing glycaemic control, particularly as **hyperglycaemia** is not always symptomatic. However, most professionals and patients recognise that abolition or reduction of diabetic symptoms, such as polydipsia, diuresis, blurred vision and fatigue is both necessary and desirable.

Recurrent **hypoglycaemia** indicates poor glycaemic control; these episodes may occur when there has been an error in dosage of blood glucose-lowering medication (usually insulin), a small or missed meal or unplanned exercise (when medication dosage has not been correctly reduced). Sometimes, there is no apparent cause for hypoglycaemia.

Alcohol consumption

Alcohol consumption is measured in units.
1 unit = 9g ethanol
        = 1 spirits measure
        = 1 glass wine
        = $1/2$pint beer.
A bottle of spirits usually contains 26 to 28 units.

As with smoking, a sensible starting point is to ask the patient. However, denial is a frequent feature of alcoholism; thus, some patients may not be entirely forthcoming about their alcohol consumption and other members of the household may prove to be better sources of information.

If the professional suspects that the patient may be drinking excessively, then a useful screening test is the CAGE questionnaire:

1. Have you ever felt you should **C**ut down on your drinking?
2. Have you ever felt **a**nnoyed at others' concerns about your drinking?
3. Have you ever felt **g**uilty about drinking?
4. Have you ever had alcohol as an **e**ye-opener in the morning?

Two or more positive answers suggest an alcohol problem exists.

Another brief screening test is the TWEAK scale[19], which has been validated for screening women and consists of five questions:

1. How many drinks does it take before you begin to feel the first effects of the alcohol? OR
1a. How many drinks does it take before the alcohol makes you fall asleep or pass out? (If "high" tolerance use 1; if "hold" tolerance use 1A)
2. Have your friends or relatives worried or complained about your drinking in the past year?
3. Do you sometimes take a drink in the morning when you first get up?
4. Are there times when you drink and afterwards you can't remember what you said or did?
5. Do you sometimes feel the need to cut down on your drinking?

To score the test, a 7-point scale is used. Positive answers to the first two questions each scores 2 points, and to the other three questions 1 point each. Negative answers score no points. The Tolerance-high question (question 1) scores 2 points if it is reported that three or more drinks are needed to feel high. The Tolerance-hold question (question 1A) scores 2 points if a respondent reports being able to hold six or more drinks. Another study suggested that cut-points of 3 or 4 are better than 2 for identifying harmful drinking or alcoholism[20].

Blood tests can sometimes be useful for screening excessive alcohol consumption: look for a raised mean corpuscular volume (MCV) on the blood count and/or raised gamma-GT on the liver function test.

Non-CHD diabetic heart disease

The gold standard for assessing either cardiomyopathy or left ventricular hypertrophy (LVH) is an echocardiogram, but primary care access to this service may not always be rapid or direct.

Clinical examination is only approximate, but an electrocardiogram (ECG) may be helpful for suggesting whether LVH might be present. There is no single ECG marker of ventricular hypertrophy. The clinician needs to consider the electrical axis, voltage, and ST wave changes. It is inadvisable to rely completely on a single marker, such as voltage, since a thin chest wall may produce a larger voltage and a thick chest wall may mask the voltage. Left ventricular hypertrophy should be suspected if the R wave in V6 is greater than 25mm or if the sum of the S wave in V1 and the R wave in V6 is greater than 35mm.

Cardiac autonomic neuropathy (CAN) is associated with a prolonged QT interval on an ECG. Evidence of autonomic neuropathy includes bradycardia in response to the Valsalva manoeuvre or on standing, an unchanged heart rate variation during deep breathing and orthostatic hypotension. These examination findings suggest the presence, but are not incontrovertible evidence, of CAN.

Microalbuminuria

Although the 'gold standard' that defines microalbuminuria is the albumin excretion rate (AER) in a timed urine sample, this method is impractical for large scale screening in the community. Various makes of semi-quantitative test strips are available, but these have wide ranges of sensitivity (51 to 100%) and specificity (21 to 100%). With a cut-off point for microalbuminuria of 2.5mg/mmol in males and 3.5mg/mmol in females, the albumin:creatinine ratio (ACR) correlated well with AER in a study of type 1 diabetics where the cut-off point for microalbuminuria is 3.5mg/mmol[21]. In a study done by the author, only 2.7% of initially negative ACR results were found to be positive for microalbuminuria on subsequent ACRs; thus, a single ACR estimation seems to have a very high negative predictive value, although a quarter of those with initially positive ACR results were subsequently screened as negative after repeated ACR estimations[22].

■ Key messages:

- Risk prediction tables, using annualised risk, often underestimate significantly cardiovascular risk in patients with diabetes.

- Despite several flaws, risk models derived from the Framingham data are currently the best way to predict cardiovascular risk in untreated patients, although the UKPDS risk engine is more "refined" tool for diabetics without evident CVD.

- Risk factors need to and can be accurately evaluated before predicting global risk.

- The methods for evaluating risk factors are usually available to primary care, but need to be applied and interpreted with proper care and attention.

- The increase in cardiovascular risk attached to any particular factor is not always matched by an equal reduction in risk if therapeutic interventions reduce or eliminate that factor.

Setting targets for reducing cardiovascular risk: global and individual factors

Global targets

After evaluating cardiovascular risk (subject to the provisos discussed in the previous chapter) and its components, a health care professional may now feel ready to implement the appropriate interventions (discussed in the next chapter) to minimise the likelihood of his patient suffering from a major cardiovascular event, particularly if that patient is at "high" risk.

However, planning should precede action and it is important for both the professional and the patient to consider and then to agree what should be the end result of all this activity, i.e. set a target. A few patients may have unrealistic expectations of what might be achieved with treatment, or may be "risk averse" (expect or wish that treatment has no adverse effects). However, most patients are pragmatic and are able to recognise that a significant reduction of elevated risk is beneficial, provided that the treatment is tolerable and safe.

All patients with existing CVD should be regarded as being at "high" risk of developing further cardiovascular disease; so it is reasonable to aim to reduce this global risk by correcting all modifiable risk factors (secondary prevention). In some guidance documents, patients without any evidence of CVD have been assigned to two contiguous risk groups on the basis of 10 year coronary risk. Higher-risk and lower-risk are defined as above and below, respectively, an agreed threshold. In recent years this threshold has been reduced from a 30% 10 year risk to a 15% 10 year risk, as recommended in the 2002 NICE guidance for treatment of blood pressure and lipids in patients with type 2 diabetes. In this group, for the purpose of primary prevention, the aim (or target) is to move an individual from the higher-risk group to the lower-risk group.

Before moving on, a few words of warning: when setting any targets, it is important not to forget that, ideally, these should be linked to a real adverse outcome (e.g. serious illness or death) in the patient and not to so-called surrogate endpoints. These endpoints are usually associated with no significant damage or systemic upset to the patient and, while they may have a correlation with a real outcome, this link is not necessarily or invariably strong. Therefore, caution must be used when trying to infer what effect changes in a measurable risk factor may have upon the risk of a significant adverse outcome occurring. It is often easy to be swayed by evidence of the beneficial effect of a drug upon a risk factor, as presented in promotional literature produced by pharmacological companies to sell their products.

Targets for individual parameters

In the new GP Contract some indicators (such as blood pressure, smoking cessation and total cholesterol), are duplicated in more than one disease framework[1]. Therefore, it could be financially advantageous to reach a target with some of the following parameters and attract double or triple payment for a single successful intervention.

Smoking status

In the perfect world, the aim is to promote and maintain the cessation of smoking. However, this aim may prove to be beyond some patients; therefore, the patient and clinician may have to settle for minimising the extent of the patient's smoking.

Dietary modification

There is no universal perfect diet for all patients with diabetes, since dietary advice must be tailored to the individual's needs and wishes. However, from the health perspective, one of the "core" goals of dietary advice must be to reduce cardiovascular risk by enabling and encouraging the individual to make eating choices that help correct adverse risk factors: dyslipidaemia, hypertension, obesity, and physical inactivity.

When reducing energy intake for weight reduction, a diet should aim to produce a daily deficit of 500 to 1,000 kcal, but not to drop below the bands of 1,200 to 1,600 kcal/day for men and of 1,000 to 1,200 kcal/day for women[2].

The other core goals of a diet for patients with diabetes should be to:
- Assist in the achieving and maintenance of blood glucose levels as frequently as possible within the normal range to minimise the risk of diabetic complications, particularly microvascular disease.
- Provide essential nutrition.

Simplistically, the aims of providing dietary advice to all patients with diabetes are to:
- Ensure that they have the required information about the type and quantity of food which they eat.
- Encourage them to make the most appropriate choices for eating, in accordance with their health needs and with their preferences, beliefs and lifestyle.

Physical activity

Most diabetics (as well as the general population) should seek to be more physically active. However, the type and level of physical activity needs to be appropriate and acceptable to the individual.

The ADA recommends[3] that an exercise programme in patients with diabetes should aim to fulfil the following criteria:
- Type of exercise: aerobic
- Frequency: three to five times per week
- Duration: 20 to 60 minutes of continuous or intermittent exercise
- Intensity: 55 to 79% of maximum heart rate (calculated as 220 minus age in years)
- Energy expenditure: modulate to achieve 700 to 2,000 calories per week.

Precautions also include proper warm up and cooling down, foot care, and adequate hydration and metabolic control[3].

In the UK, the Chief Medical Officer's recent report on physical activity recommends at least 30 minutes of moderate-intensity activity (e.g. brisk walking, cycling, swimming) on five or more days of the week for general health benefit and 45 to 60 minutes of moderate-intensity activity a day to prevent obesity in many people[4].

Obesity and weight

As discussed in previous chapters, achieving and maintaining an ideal body weight does not invariably equate with abolishing obesity. The ideal BMI is greater than 20 kg/m^2 and less than 25 kg/m^2 in whites (23 kg/m^2 in Indo-Asians). The ideal waist circumference is less than 102 cm in white men, 88 cm in white women, 90 cm in Asian-Pacific men and 80 cm in Asian-Pacific women.

Health professionals will know from bitter experience that massive and sustained weight loss is not easy to achieve. It is both practical and humane, particularly as the change has to result mainly from behavioural change, to set a target whose end point takes into account the starting point and that does not require an excessive rate of change (no more than 1 to 2 kg per month of weight loss). As patients get older, weight loss becomes progressively more difficult. A realistic target in some individuals may be to avoid further weight gain.

Blood pressure

Neither research evidence nor expert consensus has found a level of blood pressure below which treatment does not confer benefit. The target blood pressure levels currently recommended by several learned bodies do not concur, but the overall trend has been downwards over recent years. These different targets are summarised in Table 4.1:

Table 4.1: Target blood pressure levels recommended by different learned bodies or organisations

Blood pressure target (mmHg)	Learned body/Organisation	Date published
145/85	New GP Contract	2003
140/90	NICE[5]	August 2004
140/80	SIGN[6]	November 2001
140/80	National Clinical Guidelines for Type 2 Diabetes[7]	October 2002
140/80	UKPDS 36[8]	2000
130/80	American Diabetes Association[2]	January 2005
130/80 (optimal) 140/80 (acceptable)	British Hypertension Society Guidelines BHS- IV[9]	2004

Whatever target is chosen, a lower level seems sensible if target organ damage is evident. Less strict targets may be appropriate in elderly patients with limited life expectancy. As discussed later in this chapter, achieving such tight targets may not be possible in or acceptable to some patients with type 2 diabetes, despite or because of the concurrent prescribing of several agents. It should not be forgotten that any lowering of blood pressure reduces cardiovascular risk in all patients with diabetes (but to a variable extent): many studies achieved reductions of the order of 10 mmHg systolic and 5 mmHg diastolic. Thus, rather than aiming always for a fixed endpoint, an individualised target based upon the starting level of blood pressure and an achievable reduction may be more realistic and appropriate for some patients.

Serum lipids

Ideally, the aim should be to both improve and maintain lipids beyond the threshold at which there is an increased CHD risk. In 2002 the National Clinical Guidelines for Type 2 Diabetes did not recommend treatment with medication if:
1. Total cholesterol (TC) is less than 5.0 mmol/l (or LDL-C is less than 3.0 mmol/l) AND
2. Triglycerides (TG) are less than 2.3 mmol/l[10].

These recommendations concurred with the Joint British Societies' 1998 lipid targets for primary prevention in diabetics (with a 15% or greater risk of developing coronary heart disease over the next ten years) [11].

The ADA's recommended targets in 2005 do not include total cholesterol, but concentrate on lipoprotein fractions and are tighter than those of the Joint British Societies:
1. LDL-C less than 2.6 mmol/l,
2. TG less than 1.7 mmol/l, and
3. HDL-C greater than 1.1 mmol/l[2]

At the time of writing, the Joint British Societies are scheduled to publish later in 2005 their revised targets for lipid management. These will now include an HDL-C target, likely to be greater than 1.0 mmol/l, as well as targets for LDL-C and triglycerides.

As more studies in this field have published their findings, there is perhaps less divergence now than previously between British and American guidance on targets for the management of dyslipidaemia.

The new GMS contract quality outcomes framework's only current lipid target is a total cholesterol target of less than 5.0 mmol/l (although this could change when the QOF is reviewed). In light of the most recent evidence, simply achieving this target may not correct an atherogenic lipid profile, especially in high-risk patients. Primary care teams should give serious thought to setting targets of LDL-C, HDL-C and triglycerides for their high-risk patients.

However, as with raised blood pressure, a move away from the target as a fixed endpoints to a proportional improvement from any baseline may be "around the corner" for lipid management in high-risk patients. Evidence from two recent landmark studies, the MRC/BHF Heart Protection Study[12] and CARDS[13], showed improved outcomes with lipid-lowering irrespective of baseline levels. These findings may result in future recommendations (on both sides of the Atlantic) adopting a different and more aggressive approach to lipid regulation, where there would be no lower limit for intervention or for the target on LDL-cholesterol in patients with type 2 diabetes.

44

As with other risk factors, it is sensible to set less strict targets in some elderly patients with a limited life expectancy.

Glycaemic control

The targets for optimal glycaemic control are a glycosylated haemoglobin below an agreed threshold and the absence of extreme variations of blood glucose (no hypoglycaemia).

There is good evidence that good glycaemic control (an HbA1c of 7.0% or less) improves outcomes in patients with both type 1 and type 2 diabetes. Various authoritative guidelines have set different targets in the range of 6.5 to 7.5%, summarised in Table 4.2.

Table 4.2: Target glycosylated haemoglobin levels recommended by different bodies

Glycosylated haemoglobin (HbA1c in %)	Learned body/Organisation	Date published
7.4 or less	New GP Contract	2003
6.5 to 7.5	Royal College of General Practitioners/NICE[14]	September 2002
Less than 7.0	ADA[2]	January 2005

Although there is epidemiological evidence that there is no lower limit of HbA1c at which further lowering does not reduce the risk of complications, lower targets are associated with an increased risk of hypoglycaemia, particularly in patients with type 1 diabetes. Thus, the target agreed with the patient must be both a compromise and safe. In patients either at higher risk of developing or with existing cardiovascular disease and complications, a lower target HbA1c is desirable. Conversely, a higher target HbA1c may be appropriate in individuals either at "lower risk" or for whom hypoglycaemia would be catastrophic (i.e. elderly, isolated or infirm). Even in motivated and enabled patients, tight HbA1c targets are difficult to achieve. It is likely that, as much for practical as for clinical grounds, the new GP contract's target HbA1c is set at 7.4 % or less.

Alcohol

Unlike smoking, moderate alcohol consumption on a regular basis, but not in binges, is not harmful. Risk is a continuum and higher limits are controversial. "Low risk" drinking is 20 units or less per week in men and 15 units or less per week in women. Patients with diabetes should try to avoid drinking more than 3 units of alcohol in one session.

An "alternative" view of targets

The author has found thought-provoking two papers published in the same issue of the *British Medical Journal* in 2002 about the benefits of striving to achieve the targets advised by the various expert bodies and performance contracts.

In the first paper, Peter Winocour[15] sounded a cautionary note, arguing that current targets (that started as a mean) were achieved in only 50-70% in research studies, and that attaining these targets involves polypharmacy, which may lead to reduced patient concordance. However, the factors that influence concordance are complex and vary between individual patients. Both once- and twice-daily regimens are associated with better concordance, although once-daily dosing has the advantage of reducing the tablet "load". In patients known to miss medication, twice-daily dosing may result in shorter periods of sub-therapeutic medication levels[16].

Starting with the typical cardiovascular risk profile of many patients with type 2 diabetes, professionals who are aiming to achieve the recommended targets could prescribe simultaneously:
- two hypoglycaemic agents
- three antihypertensive agents
- two lipid-regulating agents and
- aspirin
– a total of eight drugs, in addition to prescribing for other medical problems. Understandably, many patients would find such a regimen unacceptable or difficult.

Also, clinical guidelines may fail to take into account the dropout rates in research studies.

Rather than the inflexible pursuit of several simultaneous "tough" targets, it is surely reasonable in some cases to set pragmatic individualised targets, in full collaboration with the patient, with the priority of improving the adverse measurement of each component.

Winocour suggested alternative targets for blood pressure control. These are shown in Table 4.3.

Table 4.3: *Targets for Certain Measurable Components of Diabetic Care (Winocour[15])*

Component	Current recommendation	Alternative recommendation: For an individual	Alternative recommendation: For the clinic
HbA1c	7.0-7.5%	**a.** 6.5% within 3 years of diagnosis, if no complications, on diet **b.** 8% 5 years after diagnosis, if complications **c.** 9% insulin treated obese	**a.** 50% < 7.5% **b.** & **c.** reduction in clinic mean by 10-20%
Blood pressure	130-140/80-85	**a.** 160/95 if aged > 75 **b.** 150/90 if CHD, microalbuminuria, dyslipidaemia or smoker **c.** Reduce BP by 10-20%	**a.** 140/90 in 40% of treated patients **b.** 160/95 in 75% of treated patients **c.** Shift clinic mean by 10-20%

In the second paper, Law and Wald[17] proposed that variables, such as blood pressure, serum cholesterol, and body mass index (discussed below), should be regarded as having a dose-response relationship with the diseases that they "cause". The authors went on to argue "that a given change in the variables reduces the risk of disease by a constant proportion of the existing risk irrespective of the starting level of the variable or existing risk."

They concluded that a patient's overall absolute level of risk, not the level of the risk factors, should determine the threshold for intervention. If a patient is assessed as carrying a high level of risk, then appropriate intervention targets should be large changes in all reversible risk factors at the same time[17].

This approach appears to be supported by the findings of the MRC/BHF Heart Protection Study that high-risk patients benefited from treatment with a statin, irrespective of the pre-treatment cholesterol level[12].

Remembering that the delivery of high quality care in this area is about reducing global cardiovascular risk, it is crucial that what is measured accurately reflects what is and should be done. It is easier to collect data about whether fixed end points have been reached (usually one measurement), than about the amount of change that has occurred (which requires an additional measurement and calculation).

To paraphrase Robert McNamara, the U.S. Secretary of Defence in the 1960s, we must avoid, "making what is measurable important, and find ways of making the important measurable".

Ultimately, it is quite possible to fail to reach a target but achieve a significant reduction in risk, particularly in an individual who starts at high risk; whereas in another individual reaching a target may result from minimal change but achieve a lesser reduction of risk.

Perhaps, the important messages to take on board from these two papers are that:
1. Targets should be set at a realistic and achievable level for the individual patient.
2. All treatable risk factors should be attacked in patients identified as "high risk".
3. Any improvement in a risk factor is likely to produce some benefit, whatever the starting point.

■ Key messages:

- In primary prevention of CVD, the target should be to reduce global risk, ideally moving the individual from the higher to the lower 10 year coronary risk group.

- As targets, reducing "hard" cardiovascular event outcomes should have priority over improving risk factors.

- An intervention target can be set for each modifiable risk factor; targets may need adjusting depending upon other factors or circumstances relating to the patient.

- For some risk factors, such as blood pressure and lipids, targets are evolving; in the future it possible that there will be no "lower limit" for intervention and/or endpoint.

- In higher-risk individuals targets need to be realistic, all factors should be attacked, and any improvements are likely to be of benefit.

Interventions to reduce cardiovascular risk

An overview of the approach to reducing risk

This chapter discusses the different interventions that may improve each of the modifiable parameters associated with cardiovascular risk. During each patient encounter, the health professional needs to consider the tackling of each specific parameter within the broader objective of reducing overall risk. Some interventions, particularly those of lifestyle modification, can improve more than one parameter.

As part of the full periodic review (usually carried out annually), cardiovascular risk should be assessed and any appropriate interventions can then be planned and implemented. Interim reviews may provide opportunities to target areas where the need for change is greatest. Additionally, if the patient presents for other conditions where diabetes may not be the priority for either the professional or the patient, cardiovascular risk reduction should not be totally overlooked. The management of some adverse risk markers may not specifically tackle the marker itself, but rather the associated factors that influence it.

The health professional who is involved in interventions that seek to alter patient behaviour needs to remain calm, patient and non-judgemental. Some patients can induce strong negative emotions in others, but the professional needs to strike the right balance between conveying empathy and displaying an appropriate professional detachment. Where a change in patient behaviour is "required", the professional needs to look beyond the prescription pad and to employ an approach based more upon health educational and psychological techniques. The professional should also try to identify and address any psychological and social factors that may affect the patient's capability to self-manage.

Crucial to a "patient-centred" approach to cardiovascular risk management is the patient's accurate understanding of this risk and how it may be affected by intervention. Effective strategies to improve this understanding need to take into account context, health beliefs and opportunities to influence risk. The 27 September 2003 issue of the British Medical Journal contains several useful articles that discuss this complex area.

The decision to alter lifestyle is "owned" by the patient and successful improved outcomes cannot be guaranteed. Change is often challenging for the patient, who may looking to the professional for a therapeutic "magic wand" (pharmacological), which may be neither available nor the mainstay of effective change. Change is also challenging for the professional, who should be prepared to invest some time and effort in order to help it happen. Professionals who become involved may need to review their conceptual thinking about illness, moving away from a biomedical model (which is very "professional-centred") to a bio-psycho-social model that encompasses the effect of the illness on the individual's functioning within his/her environment and the importance of patient choice[1]. This will apply particularly to improving lifestyle factors: smoking cessation, dietary modification, increased physical activity, weight loss and reduction of excessive alcohol consumption.

Following descriptions of available interventions, the final section of this chapter summarises the most effective ways to improve outcomes in patients with both diabetes and CHD.

The importance of health education

A personal view

Many GPs and practice nurses lack both the time and skills to provide effective health education for their patients. And yet, providing suitable advice is often an essential component of management. Most professionals do attempt to provide short bursts of "health education" in many of those consultations that deal with chronic disease. Adding up these interventions over a long period, such as a month or a year, it is highly likely that a professional would have devoted considerable time to health education. Infrequently a professional has changed a patient's behaviour with a single piece of appropriate advice. More frequent meaningful change from such interventions would both benefit patients and increase professionals' job satisfaction.

Every professional can easily create a list of the "usual suspects", regular consulters whose chronic problems are caused or exacerbated by their poor lifestyle, and who remain impervious to suggestions of modifying their behaviour, while eternally expecting the professional to provide the non-existent "miracle cure". Improving lifestyle to reduce cardiovascular risk in these individuals is a big challenge.

Patients often know more than is credited about their disease and other health matters. The priority of health education is more often to facilitate behavioural change than to simply "spoon feed" information. This requires an approach that is not didactic, but that does draw upon the working methods of educationalists and psychologists.

The author has found it useful to draw upon four overlapping concepts in a simplistic way to enhance the effectiveness of educational interventions within the consultation:
- effective consultation technique
- the educational triangle
- the trans-theoretical model of change, and
- cognitive behaviour therapy.

Effective consultation technique

Health professionals should aim to use good effective consultation behaviours in all patient contacts without slighting the necessary clinical content. Gask and Usherwood published a very succinct useful overview[2], but there is a wealth of excellent literature to guide those with an interest[3,4]. Within the consultation a professional is more likely to provide good patient care and to facilitate more optimal health behaviour in the patient if:
- the professional's core skills of clinical expertise, communication and problem-solving are organised and deployed effectively
- not just physical factors, but also emotional and social factors are considered
- the patient's agenda is addressed and the patient is involved appropriately in any decision-making process.

Educational triangle

GP trainers will recall the recognised educational triad of "aims, methods and assessment," which can also be applied to health education for patients:
1. **Aims** can address any combination of knowledge, skill or attitude "needs", as agreed by the learner and the provider.
2. **Methods** may involve a range of activities from one-on-one to groups, printed and video literature and electronic resources.
3. **Assessment** here is formative and requires repeating regularly, so as to provide the information needed to revise and prioritise the patient's educational needs.

Trans-theoretical model of change

In the 1980s the trans-theoretical model of change was published for addiction behaviours[5]. Subsequently, many professionals felt that the model could be applied to various health-related behaviours, such as smoking, alcohol consumption, diet and exercise. This model is particularly attractive because it recognises that different strategies are required to further change at each stage, and because it reflects the progress and relapses that occur in real life. The model is summarised in Table 5.1.

As can be seen, the patient thinking about change (at the contemplative stage) can be helped through the sequential stages of *preparation*, *action* and *maintenance*, hopefully with the outcome of safer or healthier behaviour. Relapses can occur but, if recognised, patients can be guided back to the preparation and action stages.

Various triggers may cause a patient to move from being unwilling to being prepared to think about change. This transformation may result from realising that an adverse event may be imminent or more likely, that the problem is connected to his current behaviour, and that the benefits of change outweigh the risks and/or disadvantages. If a patient appears unwilling to change, then the professional may wish to use one or more of the following strategies to help the patient move from the pre-contemplation to contemplation:
- emphasise the positive health and social benefits of change
- focus upon the risks of maintaining a particular unhealthy aspect of lifestyle
- help the patient to demolish or find a route around any barriers to change.

Whatever strategy is used, the professional is likely to be seeking to alter the patient's motivation at this point (as discussed in the next section).

Table 5.1: The trans-theoretical model of change

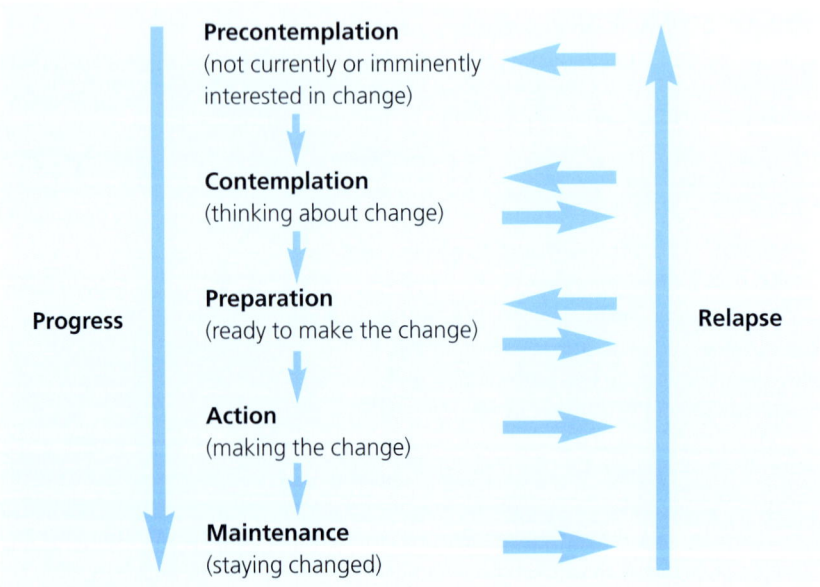

Cognitive behaviour therapy (CBT), problem solving and motivational approaches

Cognitive behaviour therapy

CBT refers to a group of psychological treatments that include behaviour therapy, behaviour modification and cognitive therapy in various combinations.

- **Behaviour approaches** aim to change behaviour, both as a therapeutic aim in its own right, and to produce other symptomatic improvements.
- **Cognitive approaches** explore how cognition mediates feelings and behaviour. Therapy aims to identify maladaptive thought patterns and to teach the patient to recognise and challenge these.

In practice, therapists combine both approaches[6].

There is now increasing interest in using CBT to modify other behaviours. GPs and nurses can apply brief focused CBT interventions that are far more likely to be effective than a "lecture", which is mainly telling the patient what to do, and which risks being counter-productive. The CBT process can be divided, broadly, into three sequential steps:

1. Baseline: "Where are you now?"
The professional aims to identify the patient's current state (behaviours, thoughts and feelings) with regard to his condition and well-being, prior to the process of goal setting.

2. Outcome: "Where do you want to get to?"
By asking the patient to define his goals and aims to assist him towards his "picture of health", the professional can help the patient to explore the benefits of change, with attention to the expected gains (physical, psychological, cognitive). Goal identification enables the patient and professional to know when the intervention is completed, thus providing momentum for change.

3. Process: "How are we going to get there?"
An agreed plan of action may include various techniques, including problem solving, graded task setting (small manageable goals that will generative greater self-confidence from success), visualisation, inter-personal "coaching", and other educational techniques. Both patient and professional will have clearly defined responsibilities in the implementation of the action plan.

When the patient reaches the second stage ("Outcome") of the CBT process, he could be regarded as being at the "contemplative stage" of the trans-theoretical model. To help a patient move through the CBT process, the professional should employ effective consulting techniques, together with motivational interviewing (summarised in Table 5.2).

Motivation

Motivation influences lifestyle and is owned by the individual. In order to better understand motivation so as to change it, the professional needs to be aware of the two main components of motivation. These include:

Importance, made up of:
- knowledge about gains and losses resulting from any particular behaviour
- concern (balance between too little and too much) about that behaviour

and

Confidence, made up of:
- self-esteem
- self-efficacy (belief in the individual's capability to act).

Structured and suitably directed information gathering by the professional will enable him to develop a greater understanding of the patient's current situation: the constructs of the patient's motivation (importance of current behaviour and his self-confidence) and an awareness of what outcomes might be feasible from a change in behaviour. Simple questions can be asked to explore importance (e.g. "How do you feel now on a scale of 1 to 10?") and confidence (e.g. "How confident on a scale of 1 to 10 do you feel about being able to change X, Y or Z?") about making a change.

Referring to the trans-theoretical model of change described above:
- at pre-contemplation the importance score will be low
- at contemplation the importance score will be high, but the confidence score may be low
- at preparation, both scores need to be high.

Identifying and stimulating the patient's awareness of the need for change can use motivational *"linguistic patterns"* to emphasise the benefits of change; e.g. "As you begin eating more healthily and regularly, you will notice that your general well-being will improve. This will be because your blood sugar is becoming stable, and this, in turn means that you will have more energy".

Where there is ambivalence about importance, a useful exercise is to ask the patient to complete a grid (this can be done away from the consultation), comparing the benefits and losses of change against those of no change. Another strategy is to explore what would need to happen or alter to increase the importance of change for the patient. It is important that the patient is "enabled" to express concerns about his current behaviour and the arguments for change, in order that his "decisional balance" is tipped towards action.

Where confidence is low, the professional needs to consider what "blocks" confidence; these may include:

- lack of knowledge and skills
- lack of support (from family, friends or professionals)
- past failures to change
- poor function (lack of alternative behaviours)
- psychological distress, such as anxiety, depression, low self-esteem.

The nature of the "block" will determine what strategy is used to try to dismantle it. It is sometimes useful to ask a patient to recall what strategies he used to achieve a previous success.

The important tasks of motivational interviewing are summarised in Table 5.2.

Table 5.2: The key tasks of motivational interviewing

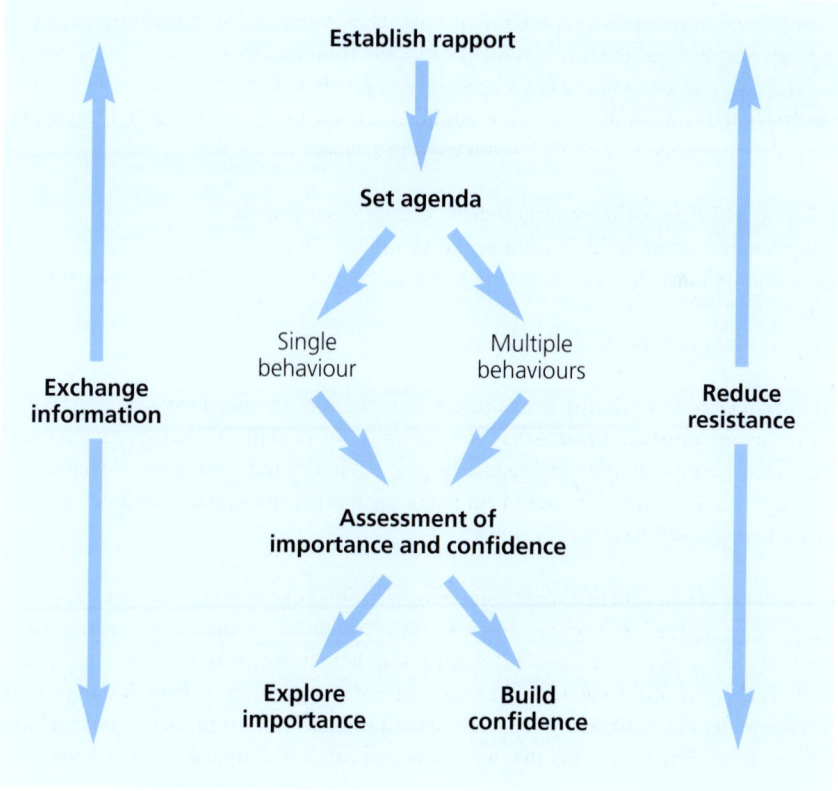

Secondary gain

In the domain of a psychological approach, the professional needs to be aware of the effects of possible secondary gain, control and emotional expression within a patient's illness behaviour.

Most people know what is beneficial for them and how to achieve it. Just as smoking cessation interventions are ineffective when the "benefits" to the patient of remaining a smoker are ignored or not accepted, so too can some features be overlooked within the psychological management of physical conditions. For example a patient who, following a row with his partner, sabotages some aspect of his diabetic programme (perhaps ignoring his diet or "forgetting" his medication), thus forcing the partner to take the roles of rescuer and consoler. This sabotage may be the means by which a patient expresses anger, but it has negative health consequences. If the professional is aware of these other features, then the professional can help the patient to recognise these issues and to identify any unconscious motives; then apply problem-solving techniques to help the patient take "ownership" of his behaviour.

Interventions to reduce global cardiovascular risk

Before considering in detail the range of interventions designed to correct the individual risk factors that combine to produce a global cardiovascular risk, it may be useful to discuss briefly another approach.

The American Diabetes Association has produced the following recommendations for the reduction of global cardiovascular risk in patients with diabetes:

1. In patients aged over 55 years, with or without hypertension, but with the presence of at least one other cardiovascular risk factor (previous history of CVD, dyslipidaemia, smoking or microalbuminuria), the prescription of an ACE inhibitor, unless contraindicated, should be considered to reduce CVD risk.

2. In patients with a previous history of myocardial infarction or undergoing major surgery, the prescription of a beta-blocker, in addition and if not contraindicated, should be considered to reduce mortality[7].

In the above circumstances the use of ACE inhibitors and/or beta-blockers should be regarded as independent from their role in the treatment of the individual risk factor hypertension (see discussion below for further details).

Due to a relative lack of interventional studies involving individuals of non-European ancestry, the effect of ethnic differences upon the efficacy of many interventions is not yet clear.

Smoking cessation

Following an evaluation to identify the potential for behavioural change and the constructs of the patient's motivation, potential interventions (discussed below) are designed to encourage and support smoking cessation and the maintenance of non-smoking behaviour.

The Cochrane Library (see also Appendix 4) has evaluated the evidence for the efficacy of various interventions to promote smoking cessation and has concluded that a variety of effective strategies are available[8]. Both nicotine replacement therapy and bupropion have been the subjects of NICE guidance[9].

Following a White Paper, the Government set up a comprehensive NHS Stop Smoking Service in 1999. This has a budget of £51,000,000 for the financial year 2005/2006[10]. In addition to the sustained and high profile public health campaigns to highlight the dangers of smoking, the Service has funded initiatives such as counselling services, a NHS Smoking Helpline[11] and the smoking cessation aids NRT and bupropion.

Advice

If the patient is prepared to consider and undertake quitting, then a reasonable initial approach may be to reinforce the benefits of smoking cessation and to advise the patient to set a date for stopping. Brief focused interventions consisting of advice given by health professionals can achieve smoking cessation rates of 2%[12].

NICE guidance for prescribing smoking cessation aids

A more detailed discussion of the smoking cessation aids, NRT and bupropion follows. In 2002 NICE published guidance about the prescription of these items[9]:
- NRT or bupropion should only be prescribed to smokers who commit to a target stop date.
- Neither NRT nor bupropion should be prescribed to smokers under the age of 18 years.
- Both NRT and bupropion should not be prescribed in combination.

- The initial prescription of NRT should provide sufficient quantities to last for two weeks after the target stop date. The initial prescription of bupropion should be sufficient to last for three to four weeks after the target stop date.
- Second prescriptions for NRT and bupropion should only be given to people who have demonstrated that their attempt to quit is being sustained when reassessed.
- If an attempt to stop smoking is unsuccessful, the NHS should not normally fund a further attempt with NRT or bupropion within six months.

Smoking cessation clinics

An increasing number of smoking cessation clinics have been set up throughout the NHS. These clinics can provide starter courses of smoking cessation aids (such as NRT and bupropion), are directly accessible to patients and are run by trained counsellors. Many practices are also running their own smoking cessation programmes. Practice nurses are ideally placed to receive the appropriate training to run these clinics. Smoking cessation clinics are more effective than brief advice or usual care in motivated "quitters".

Nicotine replacement therapy

Smoking cessation rates can be doubled in motivated "quitters" smoking more than 10 cigarettes per day, when advice is combined with nicotine replacement therapy (NRT)[13]. The available formulations of NRT include transdermal patches, chewing gum, inhalation or nasal spray for physical withdrawal symptoms, e.g. the first cigarette before breakfast (see BNF section 4.10 for further details). All forms are effective and are available either over the counter or on an NHS prescription. The dose depends upon the number of cigarettes smoked per day. NRT is fairly safe, but NICE recommends caution in patients with cardiovascular disease, hyperthyroidism, severe renal or hepatic impairment and peptic ulcer, as well as diabetes (although the dangers of continuing to smoke usually far outweigh the potential side effects of NRT). Some formulations of NRT are contra-indicated in pregnancy.

Antidepressants

The antidepressants bupropion (Zyban – see BNF section 4.10) and nortriptyline have increased smoking cessation rates in a small number of trials, independently of whether depression was present. Since patients in these trials were offered also behavioural support, these drugs are prescribed most effectively within a structured counselling programme[8].

Bupropion is available currently on NHS prescription for smoking cessation. The main adverse events associated with bupropion are seizures, which occur in about 1 in 1000 patients. In addition, it is also recommended that patients prescribed bupropion should have their blood pressure monitored, as rises have been reported, even in normotensive individuals.

Other methods of smoking cessation

Other methods that have been used for smoking cessation are considered either ineffective (anxiolytics and lobeline), of uncertain benefit (acupuncture, aversion therapy, hypnotherapy), or limited by side effects (clonidine).

As discussed below in the obesity reduction section, it is possible that the cannabinoid receptor antagonist, rimonabant, may have potential as an aid to smoking cessation.

Dietary modification

A poor diet's contribution to increased cardiovascular risk and the goals of dietary advice have been discussed in previous chapters. Dietary modification is also referred to as medical nutritional therapy (MNT).

This section concentrates upon the aspects of dietary modification that address the aim of reducing cardiovascular risk. To achieve this, dietary interventions need to focus on improving other parameters associated with cardiovascular risk, especially obesity, dyslipidaemia, and raised blood pressure. In patients with (or at risk of developing) type 2 diabetes, the cumulative effect of these interventions should be to reduce insulin resistance (see Chapter 2). As with other "lifestyle" risk factors, the main thrust of dietary modification is to alter patient behaviour, using many of the concepts discussed above.

In 2003 Diabetes UK issued a comprehensive list of consensus-based recommendations for people with diabetes that drew upon many sources to provide detailed practical advice for professionals to implement[14].

Following an assessment (as discussed in Chapter 3), specific dietary advice needs to look at helping the patient to make appropriate changes in the composition, quantity and preparation of food that he consumes. A summary of the main recommendations of the Diabetes UK report is given in Table 5.3.

Table 5.3: *Summary of recommendations for the composition of a diet for people with diabetes (from the Diabetes UK 2003 report)*

Component	Comments
Protein	• Not > 1g per kg body weight (different for nephropathy and children)
Total fat	• < 35% of energy intake
Saturated + transunsaturated fat	• < 10% of energy intake
n-6 polyunsaturated fat	• < 10% of energy intake
n-3 polyunsaturated fat	• Eat fish, especially oily fish, 1–2 times weekly • Fish oil supplements not recommended
cis-monounsaturated fat*	• 10–20%
Total carbohydrate*	• 45–60%
Sucrose	• Up to 10% of daily energy, eaten within the context of a healthy diet • Consider using non-nutritive sweeteners where appropriate if overweight and/or hypertriglyceridaemic
Fibre	• No quantitative recommendation • *Soluble fibre* has beneficial effects on glycaemic and lipid metabolism • *'Insoluble' fibre* has no direct effects on glycaemic and lipid metabolism, but its high satiety content may help weight loss and is advantageous to gastrointestinal health
Vitamins and anti-oxidants	• Encourage foods naturally rich in vitamins and antioxidants • Supplements are usually not recommended (except in special circumstances) and some may be harmful
Salt	• < 6 g sodium chloride per day

*combined should total 60–70% of energy intake

Weight management

With weight loss and stabilisation assuming a high priority in overweight diabetics, dietary interventions need to be effective and acceptable. Achieving sustained weight loss is very difficult. The best way of "maximising" success is to incorporate dietary modification into a structured programme, tailored to the patient's own needs and preferences, and including regular physical activity and regular monitoring.

To achieve the aim of losing 1 to 2 kg per month, dietary advice should be guiding and supporting the patient in eating choices that produce a sustained energy deficit of 500 kcal per day. The dietary assessment should identify where changes in dietary habits and food choices can produce a calorific deficit.

Most people eat a fairly consistent volume of food from day to day, irrespective of its energy content. A substantial reduction in total quantity is often difficult. A more effective approach is to focus upon reducing the energy content of this bulk (the dietary energy density, expressed as kcal per 100g or 100ml of food), allowing a sufficient amount of food to be consumed for satiety, but with a lower energy yield.

Probably the most important change is to replace fat-rich foods and other dietary fat sources with starchy carbohydrate foods (particularly those containing cereal fibres) and fruit and vegetables. This should be compatible with the "Balance of Good Health", discussed in Chapter 3, and with maintaining nutrition (one of the aims of dietary advice). These changes may not only contribute to weight loss, but also improve the patient's lipid profile (see below). Alcohol contains 7kcal/g, and should be restricted in a weight management programme.

Another important aspect is the pattern of meals and snacks. If the daily energy intake is appropriate, the frequency of meals is not critical; however, dieticians advise eating at regular intervals and not undergoing prolonged spells without food, thus avoiding a "feast or famine" eating pattern. By making the mealtime an occasion to enjoy and savour food, patients may avoid abstractly consuming (possibly excess quantities of) food while focussed upon another activity.

Very low calorie diets (VLCD) are defined as containing less than 800 kcal per day and are designed to produce more rapid weight loss in very obese individuals (BMI greater than 35 kg/m^2). However, there is no evidence that they produce better long-term results than a more conventional weight loss diet. Furthermore, VLCDs do not promote behavioural changes and food choices needed to maintain weight reduction, and may increase the predisposition to binge eating. VLCDs should only be used under careful specialist supervision with close attention paid to glycaemic control and nutritional maintenance.

Improving serum lipid profile

Dyslipidaemia is more likely to occur in hyperglycaemia and needs to be corrected. Dyslipidaemia associated with insulin resistance can be found in many patients with type 2 diabetes and some overweight patients with type 1 diabetes. As discussed in Chapter 2, the abnormal lipid profile in these individuals tends to show elevated serum triglyceride levels, elevated small dense LDL particles, and reduced HDL-cholesterol levels.

Total cholesterol is less important than the amount of saturated fat in the dietary intake. The most important modification required is a reduction in saturated fat, the principal dietary contributor to serum LDL-cholesterol levels. Saturated fat and transunsaturated fat should together provide less than 10% of the daily energy intake (reduced to less than 8% in some patients). If weight loss is not necessary, then energy from saturated fat should be replaced by that from carbohydrate and cis-monounsaturated and polyunsaturated fat. Sources of fatty acids are shown in Table 5.4.

Table 5.4: *Sources of Fatty Acid (from Diabetes UK report 2003)*

cis-monounsaturated	*Trans*unsaturated	*Poly*unsaturated
• Olive oil • Fat spreads derived from olive oil • Some rapeseed oils	• Hydrogenated vegetable oils (hard margarine) • Manufactured foods containing hydrogenated vegetable oils (pies, pastries, biscuits, cakes)	• *n-6* • Corn, sunflower, safflower, Soya bean oils, and seeds • Fat spreads derived from these oils • *n-3* • Oily fish and marine oils

Sterols and stanols of plant origin have been shown to reduce serum LDL-cholesterol levels, and are now incorporated into spreads and other fat-derived products, such as yoghurts, semi skimmed milk, cereal bars and soft cheeses. These are marketed as adjuncts to other methods of lowering LDL-cholesterol. However, the spreads are markedly more expensive than conventional margarines, their effect on long-term cardiovascular morbidity and mortality is unknown, and their benefits may be offset by reductions in fat-soluble vitamin absorption and in plasma concentrations of the antioxidants ß- and α- carotene and vitamin E. One spread contains significant quantities of transunsaturated fatty acids.

Hypertension

There are a number of dietary modifications that can contribute to lowering blood pressure:

- **Weight loss** in the overweight. A loss of 1kg body weight should produce a fall of 1mmHg in mean arterial pressure.

- **Salt restriction**. Reducing the daily intake from 12g to 6g can produce a fall in blood pressure of 5/2-3 mmHg. Salt restriction can potentiate the blood pressure-lowering effect of some agents in patients with type 2 diabetes. However, since most commercial cereal and bread products contain 1% salt by weight, increasing the intake of starchy carbohydrate may offset salt restriction if these products are used. The preferable alternatives are to eat unsalted cereals such as porridge and muesli, to use a home bread-maker to produce low salt or salt-free bread, and to replace some cereal foods with fruit and vegetables.

- **Reduce alcohol consumption** (see also below).

The American Dietary Approaches to Stop Hypertension (DASH) is an eating plan that advises hypertensive individuals to consume a diet rich in fruit, vegetables and low fat dairy products with a reduced content of saturated and total fat. Those who follow this diet combined with sodium restriction can expect to their lower systolic blood pressure by 8 to 14mmHg[15]. The eating plan can be easily downloaded off the internet[16].

Although there appears to be an inverse relationship between blood pressure levels and the consumption of potassium (found in fruit and vegetables), magnesium and calcium, the 2004 BHS guidelines do not recommend supplementation of these minerals.

Due to recent concerns about the accuracy of food labelling in the UK, shoppers do need to pay close attention to the information provided on labels and to not accept blindly adjectives such as "healthy", "low", "high" or "restricted".

Carbohydrate management

The glycaemic response to foods can be affected by several factors:

- The quantity of carbohydrate consumed. The amount of carbohydrate in meals or snacks has a much greater effect on glycaemia than the source or type of carbohydrate.
- The type of carbohydrate consumed (its proportional content of glucose, fructose, sucrose, lactose, amylose, amylopectin or resistant starch).

- The effects of cooking or processing on food structure.
- Other meal components (fats and proteins).

Strict carbohydrate restriction is counter-productive and no longer belongs to diabetes management. However, controlling the total carbohydrate intake is important in optimising glycaemic control, and carbohydrate counting is being taught to some patients with diabetes.

Quantity of carbohydrate

Patients on two fixed insulin injections daily will achieve better glycaemic control if the timing, quantity and source of the carbohydrate content in their diets are fairly consistent on a day to day basis. Some patients may prefer or need to have simple advice about their intake. A common and effective qualitative method of dietary advice for carbohydrate management is the "plate method", suitable for patients with type 2 diabetes either not on insulin or on insulin in fixed doses. The dinner plate serves as a pie chart to demonstrate the proportions of the plate that can be covered by the different main food groups. 1/5 of the total area (the smallest sector) is for meat, fish, eggs or cheese. 2/5 is for the staple food (rice, pasta, bread, potatoes, etc.) and 2/5 is for fruit and vegetables.

Knowledgeable patients, particularly those on insulin regimens such as basal bolus, can be taught to how to maintain reasonably stable plasma glucose levels during varying carbohydrate intake at mealtimes by adjusting insulin dose and/or level of physical activity. Educational programmes for insulin and dietary adjustment have been set up and studied in different countries. In the UK, the DAFNE project teaches adult patients with type 1 diabetes flexible insulin adjustments (in a basal bolus regimen) to match the carbohydrate in a free diet on a meal by meal basis. Carbohydrate counting was taught using portions (equivalent to 10 – 12 g carbohydrate) and the soluble insulin dose was adjusted by 1 to 3 units per portion. Improved glycaemic control and quality of life has been demonstrated, but the project requires the patient to be committed and it makes considerable demands upon professionals' time[17].

Type of carbohydrate

It is now clear that dietary sucrose does not increase plasma glucose levels more than isocaloric amounts of starch. The glycaemic index (GI) has been devised to quantify the glycaemic effect of different foods. However, different methods of food processing and preparation, and ripeness in some cases, can alter the GI. Therefore, it may be more beneficial to pay closer attention to the fat and caloric content of different foods.

Physical activity

The definition of physical activity is any skeletal muscle movement that expends energy above resting level, whereas exercise is a type of physical activity that is carried out to enhance or maintain an aspect of fitness.

Metabolic effects of exercise in diabetes

During physical activity, the whole body's oxygen consumption may increase by up to twenty-fold. To meet its energy needs during this increased activity, skeletal muscle uses, at a greatly increased rate, its own stores of glycogen and triglycerides in addition to free fatty acids, derived from the breakdown of adipose tissue triglycerides, and glucose released from the liver. The metabolic adjustments required to maintain normal blood glucose levels and preserve central nervous system function are mediated through hormones. An early increase in hepatic glucose production (mediated by a decrease in plasma insulin and the presence of glucagons) normally occurs during physical activity. Increases in plasma glucagons and catecholamines are crucial during prolonged exercise.

These adjustments are often lost in patients with type 1 diabetes. If insulin-deficient during physical activity, an excessive release of "counter-insulin" hormones may increase already high levels of glucose and ketones, and risk precipitating diabetic ketoacidosis. High levels of exogenous insulin may reduce or prevent the increased mobilisation of glucose induced by physical activity, risking hypoglycaemia. Patients with type 2 diabetes, treated by insulin or sulphonylureas, run similar risks, although hypoglycaemia

Table 5.5: *Effect of exercise upon other cardiovascular risk factors in type 2 diabetes*

Risk factor	Effect of exercise
Glycaemic control	benefits carbohydrate metabolism and insulin sensitivity
Hyperlipidaemia	reduces triglyceride rich VLDL; effects on HDL & LDL uncertain
Hypertension	reduces blood pressure, particularly when hyperinsulinaemia is present
Fibrinolysis	data lacking
Obesity	data lacking; thought to enhance weight loss, especially of intra-abdominal fat, in conjunction with dietary change
Insulin resistance	improves insulin sensitivity

appears to be less of a problem in this population, in whom physical activity may improve insulin sensitivity and improve glycaemic control. A summary of the effects of exercise upon other cardiovascular risk factors in patients with type 2 diabetes (there is very little data for type 1) is shown in Table 5.5.

Table 5.6: *Classification of physical activity intensity, based on physical activity lasting up to 60 minutes (from the ADA guidance)[18]*

Intensity	Maximal heart rate (%)*	Relative perceived exertion (RPE)**
Very light	<35	<10
Light	35 – 54	10 – 11
Moderate	55 - 69	12 – 13
Hard	70 - 89	14 - 16
Very hard	>90	17 - 19
Maximal	100	20

*Maximal heart rate = 220 – age   **Borg rating of relative perceived exertion (RPE) 6 to 20 scale

Table 5.7: *Guidelines for ensuring a diabetic's optimal glycaemic response to exercise*

1. **Metabolic control before exercise**
   a. Avoid exercise if fasting glucose levels are >14mmol/l with ketosis present, and use caution if glucose levels are >17mmol/l without ketosis present.
   b. Ingest added carbohydrate if glucose levels are <5.5mmol/l.

2. **Blood glucose monitoring before and after exercise**
   a. Identify when changes in insulin or food intake are required.
   b. Learn the glycaemic response to different exercise situations.

3. **Food intake**
   a. Consume added carbohydrate as needed to avoid hypoglycaemia.
   b. Carbohydrate should be readily available during and after exercise.

4. **Beware that sulphonylureas and insulin may cause hypoglycaemia during exercise**.
   If exercise is anticipated, then doses may need to be reduced (by up to 65% of insulin for vigorous exercise up to 45 minutes).

5. **Avoid injecting insulin into exercising areas, which increases its absorption and the risk of hypoglycaemia.**

Increased physical activity may be achieved either through an exercise programme or changes in lifestyle. A classification of physical activity intensity is summarised in Table 5.6.

To achieve maximum benefit, any advice or support for increased physical activity should take into account:
1. The current state of health and any existing problems.
2. The individual's attitude to change and any relevant social/cultural factors
3. What goals the patient wishes to achieve.

As well as eliciting details about the frequency, duration, type and intensity of physical activity, the professional should consider the attitude of the patient towards exercise, and social and cultural factors.

Evaluation of the patient prior to exercise

Prior to beginning an exercise programme, a diabetic needs to be assessed for the following:

- The presence of **coronary artery disease** (or of several cardiovascular risk factors) requires proper evaluation of the ischaemic response to exercise and the propensity to arrhythmia during exercise. An exercise electrocardiogram (ECG) may be required.
- **Peripheral neuropathy**, which may result in loss of protective sensation in the feet. Repetitive weight-bearing exercises can be traumatic to insensitive feet and can ultimately lead to ulceration and fractures. Treadmill, jogging and step exercises are not suitable in these patients, whereas, non-weight-bearing exercises, such as swimming, bicycling, arm and chair exercises, avoid this risk. Proper footwear and adequate foot care are always necessary, whatever form of exercise is undertaken (see below).
- The presence of **autonomic neuropathy** may limit an individual's capacity for physical activity and increase the risk of a sudden adverse cardiovascular event. Cardiac autonomic neuropathy (CAN) may be suggested by the presence of other disturbances in the autonomic nervous system (affecting skin, pupils, gastrointestinal and/or genitourinary systems), by a resting tachycardia (resting pulse greater than 100 beats per minute), or by orthostasis (a drop in systolic blood pressure of greater than 20mmHg when standing).
- Patients with **active retinopathy**, in particular **proliferative**, must avoid activities that increase systolic blood pressure, involve Valsalva manoeuvres or are jarring, since these types of exercise can increase substantially the risk of retinal detachment[19].
- **Peripheral arterial disease** may be suggested by an absence of peripheral arterial pulses, but can be confirmed by Doppler pressures.

Preparing for exercise

Ideally, although an exercise programme should ideally fulfil the criteria set out in Chapter 4, it needs to be enjoyable for the patient. There are several sensible recommendations that a health professional should make when counselling patients with diabetes about to undertake an exercise programme:

1. A session of physical exercise includes a proper warm-up and cool-down period.
A warm-up should consist of 5 to 10 minutes of low-intensity aerobic activity (e.g. walking, cycling), aimed at preparing the skeletal muscles, heart, and lungs for a progressive increase in exercise intensity. Following the warm-up and prior to beginning the exercise session proper, the muscles to be used during the session should be gently stretched for 5 to 10 minutes. After the session a cool-down should be structured similarly to the warm-up in order to gradually bring the heart rate down to the pre-session level.

2. During the session, the feet need to be protected against unnecessary trauma, especially if neuropathy and/or vascular impairment are present.
Proper footwear is essential:
- socks should be polyester or blend (cotton-polyester)
- silica gel or air insoles might be used to prevent blister formation, keep the feet dry, and minimise trauma.
Patients with diabetes need to be taught to monitor their feet carefully for blisters and any other damage before and after each exercise session.

3. Proper hydration needs to be maintained throughout the session to prevent dehydration, which can affect blood glucose levels and heart function.
Adequate quantities of fluids should be taken before and during (early and frequently) the exercise session to compensate for losses through sweating.

4. During exercise, optimal metabolic control needs to be maintained.
Guidance for this is provided in Table 5.7.

5. High-resistance exercise using weights is not suitable for older patients or those with long-standing diabetes.
However, moderate weight training programmes to maintain and/or develop upper body strength that involves high repetitions with light weights are suitable in nearly all patients with diabetes.

6. Some visible form of diabetes identification should be worn during exercise.

Although increased physical activity has significant benefits on other cardiovascular risk factors, it remains to be proven that it improves cardiovascular outcomes.

Obesity reduction

Overview

As with other risk factors, the most important component of the management of obesity is enabling and maintaining a change in the patient's behaviour. There needs to be a reversal in the imbalance between a usually excessive dietary calorific intake and an inadequate level of physical activity. As discussed in Chapter 4, the target weight and rate of loss (ideally 1 to 2 kg per month) need to be negotiated. Dietary modification and increasing physical activity are discussed in greater detail above in this chapter. When weight loss is an important on-going activity for the patient, more frequent reviews may be needed to monitor progress and to encourage the patient. Specialist help should be sought if the patient is very obese or fails to respond to medical interventions.

Anti-obesity drugs

Anti-obesity agents may help diabetics to lose weight when prescribed in combination with a restricted energy diet and, ideally, increased physical activity. There are two main agents in current use, orlistat and sibutramine, which act by different mechanisms, and which have been shown to produce clinically significant weight loss in patients with type 2 diabetes, including those treated with sulphonylureas. Both are expensive and have been the subject of technology appraisals by NICE.

1. **Orlistat** acts within the stomach and small intestine as a long-acting inhibitor of pancreatic lipases. Its mode of action is to prevent the hydrolysis and subsequent absorption of ingested dietary fat (about 30%). The current prescribing licence for orlistat allows it to be prescribed to diabetes aged 18 to 75 years with a BMI of 28 kg/m² or more, who can adhere to a hypocaloric diet, losing at least 2.5kg in weight in the month prior to initiating treatment. Treatment with orlistat can be continued up to 12 months (occasionally up to 24 months), provided that a further 5% of body weight is lost by the end of three months' treatment and 10% by the end of six months[20]. Orlistat's main side effect is faecal incontinence.

2. **Sibutramine** has a different mechanism of action. It is an anorectic agent that acts centrally by inhibiting serotonin and noradrenaline reuptake, resulting in enhanced satiety. Patients will feel satisfied with smaller food portions. Sibutramine has several important contra-indications (important macro- and micro-vascular disease, uncontrolled hypertension, severe renal impairment, glaucoma, benign prostatic hypertrophy with urinary retention) and it interacts with a number of other drugs, including antidepressants, drugs affecting CYP3A4 or serotonin levels. Sibutramine

can be prescribed to diabetics aged 18 to 65 years with a BMI of 27 kg/m[2] or more. Continuation beyond the first 4 weeks requires a weight loss of 2kg; while continuation beyond 3 months requires a loss of 5% of the initial weight at the start of treatment. The maximum duration of treatment in the licence is 12 months[21].

Other therapeutic strategies to tackle obesity are being explored. A possible addition to the formulary is in phase III trials at the time of writing. Rimonabant (proprietary name Acomplia) is a central cannabinoid (CB1) receptor antagonist that suppresses appetite. It also shows promise in assisting smoking cessation. Data from early trials is encouraging with significant improvement in several cardiovascular risk factors, but 1 in 8 study subjects had to withdraw due to its side effects, which include depression, anxiety and nausea[22]. Caution is urged because this drug targets the endocannabinoid system, which regulates pleasure, relaxation and pain tolerance; its long-term effects need to be carefully evaluated and could be significant.

Gastric reduction (bariatric) surgery

The use of surgery to limit food intake and produce long term weight loss is a radical and costly approach to reduce obesity. Several surgical techniques are now available and have been studied. These include jejuno-ileal bypass, vertical banded gastroplasty and gastric bypass, all of which can result in significant weight loss. The more invasive the surgery, the greater the associated mortality and morbidity, but severe obesity also carries significant risk.

Gastric reduction can now be performed laparoscopically (using an adjustable LAP-BAND). It can produce substantial and sustained weight loss in patients with a BMI greater than 35 kg/m[2]. It does appear to improve some of the major cardiovascular risk factors[23], but there is no current data to compare the long-term benefits and risks of surgery with medical management in patients with diabetes. In a severely obese non-diabetic population, the Swedish Obese Subjects Study reported improvements in lifestyle (lower energy intake and increased physical activity), hypertension and some biochemical variables (lower triglycerides and uric acid, but not hypercholesterolaemia) in those who underwent gastric surgery, compared to those who received conventional medical treatment[24].

Blood pressure reduction

Two sources of expert guidance for the management of raised blood pressure were published in 2004:

1. British Hypertension Society Guidelines BHS- IV[25], and
2. NICE's guidance was produced by the North of England Hypertension Guidance Development Group[26].

Although both of these guidelines are not aimed primarily at a diabetic population, they are thorough, authoritative and quite relevant to the management of raised blood pressure in patients with diabetes. The management of raised blood pressure in patients with diabetes can be based sensibly and mainly upon the guidance provided by these two documents.

However, observant readers will note that the recommendations given by different expert bodies for the level of blood pressure above which medication should be started is not consistent. This inconsistency may be due to not only different target blood pressures (see Table 4.1), but also due to a gap between the threshold and the target for treatment in some guidance. Such differences or gaps are illustrated in the two following examples found in widely disseminated guidelines:

● The NICE guidelines produced in 2002 to support the publication of the National Service Framework (NSF) for Diabetes and in 2004 for hypertension did **not** recommend the prescription of medication to patients with type 2 diabetes with a blood pressure between 140/80 and 160/100, but having been designated as "low" coronary event risk.

● The British Hypertension Society 2004 Guidelines (BHS-IV) recommends initiating treatment if blood pressure is sustained at or above 140/90 in patients with diabetes. This threshold for treatment is **above** the target blood pressure of 130-140/80.

On the other hand, the American Diabetic Association in 2005 recommends pharmacological treatment if blood pressure remains persistently above the target of 130/80 after a trial of non-pharmacological measures.

Without replaying the arguments made elsewhere in this book, all patients with diabetes should be regarded as being at **higher** risk of having a cardiovascular event. Therefore, the author finds the American approach both simpler and more logical: blood pressure persistently above target normally requires lowering by any available suitable means.

It is useful to divide the interventions for lowering blood pressure into non-pharmacological and pharmacological methods.

Non-pharmacological methods of lowering blood pressure

The non-pharmacological methods that should form an integral part of a blood pressure-lowering strategy are of no surprise and are nicely summarised in the BHS-IV guidelines published in 2004:

- Weight reduction (achieve and maintain ideal body mass index- 20 to 25 kg/m²; 20 to 23 kg/m² in Indo-Asians). The loss of 1kg body weight should result in a decrease of 1mmHg in mean arterial blood pressure.
- Regular exercise (aerobic exercise for 20 to 60 minutes, 3 to 5 times per week) can reduce systolic blood pressure by up to 4 to 9mmHg.
- Reduced alcohol intake (below the standard upper limits of 21 units per week for men and 14 units per week for women) can reduce systolic blood pressure by up to 2 to 4mmHg.
- Avoiding excess caffeine (no more than 5 cups of coffee per day)
- Restricting dietary sodium (see above) can reduce systolic blood pressure by up to 2 to 8mmHg. Hypertension in blacks is usually quite sensitive to dietary salt restriction.
- Smoking cessation.

None of the above individually will produce dramatic falls in blood pressure, but the combination may produce a sufficient fall to reduce the amount of medication required, and also help to correct other abnormal risk factors, such as dyslipidaemia and obesity. However, it is important to remember that so far no well-controlled studies have been published on the effects of diet and exercise upon hypertension in patients with diabetes.

Classes of drugs that lower blood pressure

Five classes of blood pressure lowering drugs have been shown to be effective in reducing cardiovascular mortality and morbidity in patients with type 2 diabetes and raised blood pressure:

1. Angiotensin converting enzyme (ACE) inhibitors
2. Angiotensin II receptor antagonists (ARB)
3. Beta blockers
4. Non-dihydropyridine and long-acting dihydropyridine calcium channel blockers (CCB), and
5. Thiazide and thiazide-like diuretics[7].

In addition, there are three other drug classes of blood pressure lowering drugs that are sometimes used in patients with diabetes:

6. Alpha-1 adrenergic blockers,
7. Potassium-retaining diuretics, and
8. Other antihypertensive agents (the rest).

Further details of the names and dosages of different blood pressure-lowering agents are given in Appendix 1.

Angiotensin converting enzyme (ACE) inhibitors

This class of drugs blocks the conversion of angiotensin-I to angiotensin-II (a powerful vasoconstrictor and an indirect facilitator of the sympathetic nervous system) by inhibiting the angiotensin converting enzyme. This produces a reduction in angiotensin-II levels, leading to arteriolar and venous dilatation and a fall in blood pressure.

Angiotensin-II also has other actions that are thought to be harmful to the cardiovascular system, contributing to the pathogenesis of large and small vessel structural changes in hypertension and other CVD[27]. ACE inhibitors also suppress aldosterone secretion, increase renal blood flow (producing natriuresis) and increase circulating levels of bradykinin, a powerful vasodilating cytokine which can cause cough. ACE inhibitors have little effect upon heart rate or airways resistance. The antihypertensive effect of ACE inhibitors is dose-related.

Side effects include a persistent cough in 10 to 20% of users, angio-oedema in about 1% (occurs in 4% of Afro-Caribbean users), taste disturbance and rash. Initiating an ACE inhibitor can produce a sharp fall in blood pressure in patients when the renin-angiotensin system is activated (dehydration, heart failure, accelerated hypertension), but is rarely seen in uncomplicated hypertension. ACE inhibitors should be avoided in women likely to become pregnant, due to the teratogenic risk of foetal renal maldevelopment, and in patients with bilateral renal artery disease, as this might precipitate deterioration in renal function leading to renal failure. Renal artery stenosis can be detected sometimes by listening for a renal artery bruit. Often it is sub-clinical and a routine estimation of serum creatinine within 1 to 2 weeks of initiating an ACE inhibitor will detect any deterioration in renal function early enough to stop the drug and prevent significant irreversible deterioration. The concurrent prescribing of ACE inhibitors with potassium supplements or potassium-sparing diuretics should be avoided, unless specifically required (needs careful monitoring of electrolytes).

Drugs in this class have generic names ending in "-pril". They include captopril, cilazapril, enalapril, fosinopril, imidapril, lisinopril, moexipril, quinopril, perindopril, quinapril, ramipril and trandolapril.

Angiotensin II receptor antagonists (ARB)

This class of drugs blocks type I angiotensin-II (AT1) receptors. As with ACE inhibitors, this leads to a fall in angiotensin-II levels, with resulting vasodilatation and a fall in blood pressure. These drugs are less likely than ACE inhibitors to cause cough or angio-oedema, due to their selectivity for the AT1 receptor and their lack of potentiation of bradykinin and possibly other vasopeptides. Therefore, an ARB may be suitable for patients in whom ACE inhibitors are not tolerated. Cautions and contraindications are the same as for ACE inhibitors.

Drugs in this class have generic names ending in "-sartan". Currently available are candesartan, eprosartan, irbesartan, losartan, olmesartan, telmisartan and valsartan.

Beta (ß) blockers

The antihypertensive effect of beta-blockers is not completely understood. β1-blockers competitively inhibit β-adrenoreceptors in the heart. β2-blockers inhibit β-adrenoreceptors in peripheral vasculature, bronchi, pancreas, kidneys and liver. Beta-blockers decrease the heart rate (negative chronotropic effect), the force of cardiac muscle contraction and cardiac output (negative inotropic effect), and renin secretion. It is possible that some β-blockers may have direct CNS activity, although this may not be responsible for their blood pressure-lowering effect.

The various β-blockers now available have differences in duration of action, selectivity for β1- receptors, lipid solubility and partial agonist activity (also known as intrinsic sympathomimetic activity or ISA). Drugs with ISA can stimulate as well as block adrenergic receptors. These differences make this drug class more heterogeneous than other blood pressure-lowering drug classes, and also more difficult to classify. In recent years, β-blockers have been used to treat heart failure, in addition to their established role in the manangement of hypertension and angina.

The first generation β-blockers (e.g. propranolol and oxprenolol) are generally non-cardioselective (for β1-receptors), and may produce peripheral ischaemia, CNS disturbances (e.g. lethargy, impaired concentration and memory, vivid dreams) and/or bronchospasm. These first generation drugs can also exacerbate congestive cardiac failure, reduce exercise tolerance and exacerbate metabolic abnormalities (increased triglyceride and reduced HDL-cholesterol levels, and reduced hepatic glucose mobilisation, especially when combined with thiazide diuretics).

The second generation β-blockers (e.g. atenolol, bisoprolol and metoprolol) tend to be more cardioselective and to have a less (but still demonstrable) adverse effect upon serum triglyceride and HDL-cholesterol levels.

The third generation ß-blockers (e.g. celiprolol and nebivolol) have a peripheral vasodilating effect and are not thought to have an adverse effect upon plasma lipids.

The cardiac remodelling effects of sympathetic nervous system dysfunction in the heart (see Chapter 2) may be prevented or minimised by the use of ß-blockers, especially third generation agents such as carvedilol. In heart failure trials this action may be responsible for the reduction in morbidity and mortality in patients with diabetes.

Beta blockers with ISA (e.g. acebutolol, oxprenolol and pindolol), similarly to the more cardioselective ß-blockers, are less likely to cause peripheral vasoconstriction and have lesser negative chronotropic and ionotropic effects. Low lipid-soluble ß-blockers (e.g. atenolol) are less likely to cross the blood-brain barrier and cause CNS side effects. Combined receptor antagonists (e.g. carvedilol and labetalol) act on both α- and ß-receptors. The α-blocking activity offsets peripheral vasoconstriction and the adverse effect on plasma lipids produced by ß-blockade. Non-cardioselective ß-blockers should be avoided in patients with obstructive airways disease (asthma) and/or with diabetes treated by insulin (risk of masking the symptoms of imminent hypoglycaemia). ß-blockers can also cause erectile dysfunction.

Recently, doubts have been cast on whether the ß-blocker atenolol has any effect on reducing cardiovascular mortality and stroke in patients with hypertension, despite the drug's proven blood pressure-lowering effect[28]. Because atenolol has been used as a reference drug in many studies, it is unclear whether these reservations apply to atenolol alone or to other ß-blockers as well. However, it is premature to draw any definitive conclusions and readers need to remember that:

- Blood pressure-lowering still matters and several large studies have proved that lower levels correlate with better cardiovascular outcomes, irrespective of the initial drug class used.
- Drug combinations often including ß-blockers are frequently required to achieve target blood pressure levels.
- ß-blockers have had and continue to have an important role in the management of angina and heart failure, important cardiological conditions frequently present in patients with diabetes.

Drugs in this class have generic names ending in "-lol". Other currently available ß-blockers not mentioned above include esmolol, nadolol, and timolol.

Calcium channel blockers (CCB)

This group of drugs blocks voltage-dependent calcium channels on the surface of cell membranes, preventing the influx of calcium ions into the cell and reducing the availability of intracellular calcium for muscle contraction; this leads to a reduction in vascular tone and a decrease in peripheral vascular resistance. Thus, blood pressure falls. Of the six known types of calcium channel in the cardiovascular system, the most important one is the long-lasting (L-type) channel, found in all excitable cells, including the vasculature, myocardium and cardiac conducting tissue. L-type CCBs can be subdivided into three different classes:

- **Class I, phenylalkylamines** (e.g. verapamil). They depress cardiac conduction and may precipitate heart failure if there is AV or SA node dysfunction or if prescribed concurrently with ß-blockers. Verapamil has an additional anti-arrhythmic action.
- **Class II, dihydropyridines**, abbreviated as DCCB (e.g. amlodipine, felodipine, isradipine, lacidipine, lercanidipine, nicardipine, nifedipine and nisoldipine). They are relatively selective for the blocking L-type channels in smooth muscle cells, thus inducing vascular relaxation with a fall in vascular resistance and arterial pressure. They do not depress conduction or contractility; thus, they are much less likely to precipitate heart failure. They may be used safely in combination with ß-blockers. The main side effects of DCCBs are vasodilator: dose-dependant peripheral oedema (resulting from transudation of fluid from vascular compartments into the dependent tissues due to pre-capillary arteriolar dilatation), headache, flushing, palpitations and gum hypertrophy. These side effects can sometimes be offset by dose titration or by the use of slow-release or long-acting drugs such as amlodipine, lacidipine or lercanidipine.
- **Class III, benzothiazepines** (e.g. diltiazem). This class has a slightly negative or negligible ionotropic effect.

Both class I and III CCBs are sometimes referred to as non-dihydropyridine CCBs. All three CCB classes do not affect plasma lipids or glucose metabolism, and are effective in elderly and black patients.

Bioavailability is an important factor to consider when prescribing sustained-release preparations of CCBs. Different preparations containing the same quantity of a given drug are unlikely to have identical pharmacokinetic profiles. It is recommended that such preparations are prescribed by their proprietary name and that patients are not transferred to another preparation without assessment and titration.

There is currently some debate about the efficacy and safety of CCBs. A recent prospective randomised, blinded trial suggested that ACE inhibitors were more effective than CCBs at preventing myocardial infarction in hypertensive patients with diabetes and concerns were raised over the safety of CCBs[29]. The British Hypertension Society did not support these concerns in their 1999 guidelines[30]. At the European Society of Cardiology meeting in August 2000, Furberg and his colleagues presented their meta-analysis of several trials, finding no difference in the blood pressure levels achieved by CCBs and other drug classes, but suggesting that patients receiving CCBs were at increased risk from certain major cardiovascular events (a question of safety or of efficacy?). The National Clinical Guidelines for Type 2 Diabetes in 2002 recommended prescribing long-acting (avoid short-acting) CCBs only as second-line treatment or as part of combination therapy[31]. Publication of results from large trials currently in progress should clarify matters.

Thiazide/thiazide-like diuretics

The mechanisms by which thiazide or thiazide-like diuretics lower blood pressure are complex. Their antihypertensive effect is thought to be mediated by arteriolar vasodilatation. This is partly due to the urinary loss of sodium that results from a blockade of renal tubular reabsorption of sodium. Reflex vasoconstrictor activation (including the renin-angiotensin-aldosterone system) may accompany the early loss in blood volume induced by thiazides, resulting in a temporary increase in peripheral resistance. However, following initiation of a thiazide, further blood pressure lowering will occur over a period of days as peripheral resistance gradually decreases. The antihypertensive dose-response to thiazides is flat; thus, they should be prescribed at the lowest effective dose. The duration of diuresis is not the duration of antihypertensive effect.

Thiazide diuretics include bendroflumethiazide, chlorthiazide, cyclopenthiazide, hydrochlorothiazide, hydroflumethiazide and polythiazide (generic drug names end in "-thiazide"). They may differ from thiazide-like diuretics (these include chlortalidone and indapamide) in their duration of action, ion calcium-blocking activity, and carbonic anhydrase inhibitory activity. The significance of these differences is not certain.

Although thiazide and thiazide-like diuretics are generally well tolerated and can enhance the blood pressure-lowering effect of other drug classes, they can be associated with several unwanted metabolic effects, including:
- hypokalaemia (drug and dose dependent), which requires regular monitoring of electrolytes
- worsening glucose tolerance (particularly when prescribed in combination with a ß- blocker)
- a small worsening of serum lipid profile (rises in LDL-C and triglycerides)
- a small rise in serum urate levels (avoid in gout)
- hypercalcaemia.

They can also cause erectile dysfunction, and also interact with non-steroidal anti-inflammatory drugs (less effect on blood pressure-lowering) and lithium (increased risk of lithium toxicity).

The thiazide-related diuretic indapamide appears to have a relatively neutral effect upon lipid and glucose levels, when compared to thiazides, although hypokalaemia is still possible.

Alpha (α)-1 adrenergic blockers

This class of drugs can be sub-divided into selective (e.g. doxazosin, indoramin, prazosin and terazosin) and non-selective (phentolamine). These drugs block the activation of post-synaptic α-1 adrenoreceptors in the vasculature, resulting in arteriolar and venous vasodilatation. The selective α-1 blockers do not affect glucose tolerance, uric acid and potassium levels; furthermore, they appear to improve lipid profiles by reducing total cholesterol and triglycerides, while increasing HDL-C.

The major side effects of α-1 blockers are first dose syncope and orthostatic hypotension. These effects can be minimised or prevented by prescribing a low initial dose and by avoiding concomitant prescribing of diuretics. Alpha-1 blockers should be used with caution in the elderly, as the above side effects may increase the risk of falls. The short-acting prazosin, one of the earlier members of this class, is more likely to cause postural hypotension than the longer-acting doxazosin or terazosin. Other side effects of α-1 blockers include fatigue, weakness, stuffy nose and headache.

These drugs may alleviate the symptoms of benign prostatic hypertrophy in men, particularly if there is detrusor hyperactivity, but can exacerbate stress incontinence in women.

Potassium-retaining diuretics/aldosterone antagonists

These potassium-retaining diuretics act by blocking sodium/potassium exchange in the renal distal tubules. They have two main roles in blood pressure lowering:

1. They may limit potassium loss in patients treated with thiazide or thiazide-like diuretics.
2. Spironolactone can be useful in patients with "resistant" hypertension in whom blood pressure levels may be dependent on hyperaldosteronism[32].

They should be used as add-on therapy and not as first-line diuretics, except when hyperaldosteronism has been diagnosed.

They need to be prescribed with great care in patients with impaired renal function due to the risk of hyperkalamia, particularly if combined with either an ACE inhibitor or ARB. Spironolactone can commonly cause gynaecomastia due to its anti-androgen effect.

Loop diuretics should not be prescribed for blood pressure-lowering, except in patients with impaired renal function and/or heart failure.

Centrally acting, older and other antihypertensive agents

Once a mainstay in blood pressure-lowering treatment, centrally acting, older and other antihypertensive drugs are currently reserved for patients whose raised blood pressure is not controlled by or who have contra-indications to the other drug classes. These agents are less favoured than other drug groups because side effects can be more frequent, and may be unpleasant or potentially dangerous.

These drugs include:

1. **Sympatholytic agents**, which can be subdivided into:
   - The imidazoline (I1) agonist, moxonidine, which binds highly selectively to imidazoline receptors in the brain's venterolateral medulla, causing reduced peripheral sympathetic activity. This leads to falls in peripheral resistance and blood pressure. Moxonidine has little effect on α-2 receptors, which cause dry mouth and sedation.
   - The central α-agonists, methyldopa and clonidine, reduce sympathetic vasoconstriction and total peripheral vascular resistance. The major side effects of these drugs are dose-related: sedation and drowsiness.

2. **The vasodilators**, hydralazine, diazoxide and minoxidil, act by relaxing vascular smooth muscle, producing decreased peripheral vascular resistance. Their major side effects include gastrointestinal upset and fluid retention. Minoxidil may cause hirsutism, an effect exploited by its topical use in balding men.

3. **The adrenergic neurone blocker guanethidine** acts by preventing noradrenaline release in response to sympathetic stimulation. Its side effects include orthostatic hypotension, fluid retention, bradycardia and diarrhoea.

Choosing the most appropriate drug class to initiate therapy

In this section, the cited trials are referred to by their acronyms, with their full names given in Appendix 5.

When reviewing evidence, it is crucial for the reader to distinguish between "surrogate" endpoints of levels of blood pressure achieved and the "real" endpoints of mortality or morbidity. It is also important to remember that the characteristics and treatments of subjects recruited into these trials do not always resemble the real-life patients for whom health care professionals need to make treatment decisions.

There is now substantial evidence to support the use of five of the drug classes in reducing blood pressure and cardiovascular risk in patients with diabetes and raised blood pressure. Although some data is derived from trials comparing treatments against placebo, more data is now available comapring different effective treatments or combinations. An overview of this evidence is found in Table 5.8.

As mentioned above, two studies (ABCD and FACET) have suggested that ACE inhibitors are superior to DCCB in reducing cardiovascular events in patients with type 2 diabetes[29,33]. However, in another more recent study, patients with CHD and hypertension (even in the diabetic subgroup) had a similar reduction in CVD mortality if treated with either verapamil or a ß-blocker[34]. ACE inhibitors have been shown to improve cardiovascular outcomes in high cardiovascular risk patients with diabetes, independent of whether hypertension was present[35,36]. In another study, an ARB was superior to a ß-blocker in improving CVD outcomes in a subset of patients with diabetes, hypertension and left ventricular hypertrophy[37]. The wider cardio-protective benefits of ACE inhibition seem to favour initial treatment with an ACE inhibitor or ARB, all other things being equal and in the absence of contra-indications. These drugs appear to have theoretical advantages over others by virtue of their mode of action.

In patients with diabetes and incipient or established heart failure, blockade of the renin-angiotensin and of the cardiac sympathetic nervous systems with ACE inhibitors and ß-blockers, respectively, improves outcomes. The cardioprotective effects of these drug classes should be taken into consideration when selecting a blood pressure-lowering agent.

In the BHS-IV template (discussed in more detail below), the reasoning underpinning drug selection (with the initial drug classes used from the five listed above) is that hypertension can be classified as "high renin" and "low renin" and, as such, it is best treated initially with drugs that either inhibit the renin-angiotensin system (ACE/ARB or ß-blockers – known as A or B drugs) or those that do not inhibit the renin-angiotensin system (CCB or thiazide diuretic – known as C or D drugs). "Younger" people (aged 55 years or less) and Caucasians tend to have higher renin levels in comparison to older people and blacks. Thus, the BHS would recommend initial therapy in the former group with a drug from the A or B group and in the latter group with a drug from the C or D group (see Table 5.9).

However, the BHS-IV guidance is partly contradicted by the NICE 2004 guidance, which states that there is no compelling evidence to support the opinion that different classes of drug are more effective in lowering the risk of developing cardiovascular disease in either older or younger age patients.

Table 5.8: Summary of studies of antihypertensive therapies in type 2 diabetes

Study	Description	Outcome	Diabetes sample size
ABCD	Enalapril vs. nisoldipine	Greater MI event + mortality with nisoldipine	470
ALLHAT	Chlortalidone vs lisinopril, amlodipine	Thiazides prevented more CVD (1 or more forms)	15,297
ASCOT	Amlodipine +/- perindopril vs. atenolol +/- bendroflumethiazide +/- doxazosin	Amlodipine +/- perindopril more effective in reducing stroke, all cardiovascular events, and cardiovascular mortality	2,532
CAPP	Captopril vs. ß-blocker or diuretic	Captopril group had fewer MI + lower mortality	572
FACET	Fosinopril vs. amlodipine	Both treatments reduced BP but fewer events on fosinopril	380
HDFP	Stepped care vs. referred care	More active treatment reduced total CVD + mortality	772
HOPE	Ramipril vs. placebo	Ramipril prevented events + mortality	3,577
HOT	Felodipine + other agents to target diastolic BP < 90, < 85, < 80 mmHg	Lower BP produced greatest reduction in CVD events	1,501
LIFE	Losartan vs. atenolol	Losartan prevented more CVD mortality + events	1,195
NORDIL	Diltiazem vs. ß-blocker or diuretic	Similar efficacy	727
SHEP	Chlortalidone vs. placebo	Chortalidone prevented more events and reduced total mortality	583
STOP-2	ACE vs. CCB vs. conventional treatment	Similar efficacy	719
SYST-EUR	Nitrendipine vs. placebo	Treatment reduced CVD + mortality	492
SYST-CHINA	Nitrendipine vs. placebo	Treatment reduced CVD	98
UKPDS	Captopril vs. atenolol	Similar efficacy	758

Should ethnicity be a factor in the choice of therapy? Blood pressure in blacks often responds well to dietary salt restriction and there are theoretical reasons why thiazides and CCBs may be more effective in lowering blood pressure than ß-blockers, ACE or ARB. However, a recent review concluded that "there is insufficient evidence that any antihypertensive drug or drug combination is superior in reducing morbidity and mortality outcomes in hypertensive black people[38]." There is also no evidence currently available to show that South Asians respond differently from white Europeans to blood pressure-lowering medication. The key message is that there is strong evidence that blood pressure-lowering therapy reduces cardiovascular risk in both white and non-white populations[39].

It is important to recognise that many patients with diabetes and hypertension will require combinations of drugs to achieve their target blood pressures. The reader should bear in mind the findings of three studies:
1. The UKPDS showed that captopril (an ACE inhibitor) and atenolol (a beta blocker) were equally effective in reducing the incidence of diabetic complications, with the actual level of blood pressure reduction achieved being the more important factor[40].
2. The ALLHAT (antihypertensive and lipid lowering to prevent heart attack trial) study found no large differences between initial therapy with either a chlortalidone, lisinopril and amlodipine in reducing blood pressure and cardiovascular events[41], notwithstanding certain concerns about the trial's design and conclusions.
3. The Blood Pressure Lowering Treatment Trialists' Collaboration conducted a meta-analysis of 29 trials that involved 162,341 participants with over 700,000 years of follow-up and found that "the main driver from BP-lowering therapy is BP lowering *per se*[42]."

In view of the mixed messages above, it seems sensible to select – as first-line therapy – a drug from one of the five classes of blood pressure-lowering drugs that have been shown to reduce cardiovascular mortality and morbidity in patients with type 2 diabetes and raised blood pressure. Thus, the choice should be from an ACE inhibitor, an ARB, a beta blocker, a non-dihydropiridine or long-acting DCCB, or a thiazide diuretic.

As discussed further in the next section of this chapter, treatment of hypertension in patients with type 2 diabetes, probably up to the age of 75 years, should normally be accompanied by lipid-lowering with a statin, irrespective of baseline lipid levels.

Combining drug groups

Although a large formulary of potent drugs is available, control of blood pressure can be sub-optimal. In many patients, more than one blood pressure-lowering drug needs to be prescribed concurrently to achieve target or produce a substantial reduction in blood pressure. Several factors may influence the selection of the second or third (or even fourth) drug in the combination. These include tolerability, potential drug interactions, and contra-indications.

The British Hypertension Society 2004 Guidelines produced a treatment template to assist practitioners to combine different drug classes in a rational and effective way, shown in Table 5.9. Ultimately, the "bottom line" should be to achieve the best possible blood pressure control at the expense of minimal and tolerable side effects, within the overall strategy of optimising all relevant cardiovascular risk factors.

Table 5.9: *The BHS recommendations (2004) for combining blood pressure lowering drugs*

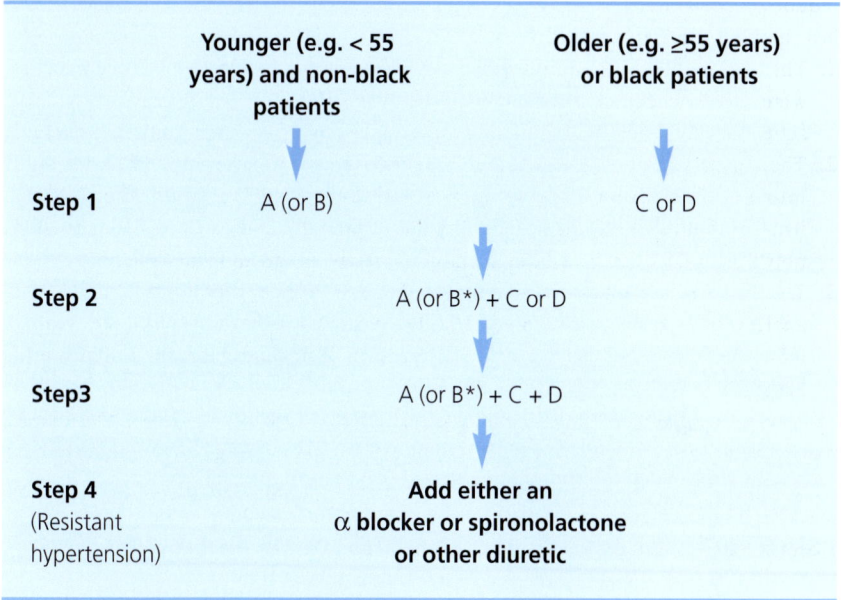

	Younger (e.g. < 55 years) and non-black patients	Older (e.g. ≥55 years) or black patients
Step 1	A (or B)	C or D
Step 2		A (or B*) + C or D
Step3		A (or B*) + C + D
Step 4 (Resistant hypertension)		Add either an α blocker or spironolactone or other diuretic

Key:
A = ACE inhibitor or ARB   B = beta blocker   C = calcium channel blocker   D = diuretic (thiazide)

*Combination therapy involving B and D may induce more new-onset diabetes (or worsen diabetic control) when compared to other combination therapies.

The blood-pressure lowering arm of the large ASCOT trial reported in September 2005[43], showing a statistically significant reduction in most of its secondary endpoints, including total cardiovascular events (absolute risk reduction 1.1%, numbers needed to treat 91), stroke (ARR 1.0%, NNT 100) and all-cause mortality (ARR 0.8%, NNT 125), using the combination of amlodipine +/- perindopril (A + C), as compared to the combination of atenolol +/- bendroflumethiazide (B + D). Some of these differences could be attributed to the lower blood pressure levels achieved and improvements in other cardiovascular risk factors (in particular, higher HDL-C) in the A + C group (both statistically significant). However, the trial lacked sufficient power to detect a statistically significant difference between the groups for the primary endpoint (non-fatal MI or CHD death). It remains to be seen precisely how this trial will influence clinical guidance and practice.

Improving serum lipid profile

The National Clinical Guidelines for Type 2 Diabetes[44] published in 2002 advised on the management of "abnormal" serum lipids. As in the management of raised blood pressure, the reduction of serum lipids can be divided into pharmacological and non-pharmacological methods.

In the 2002 National Clinical Guidelines, the previous recommendation of a threshold of a 30% risk of developing a coronary event over ten years for pharmacological intervention was reduced to 15%. A summary of the latest recommendations, which include the division of 10-year coronary event risk into higher and lower (than 15%), is set out in Table 5.10[44].

As with the blood pressure recommendations, these guidelines are not entirely logical or clearly set out. Furthermore, they pre-date the most recent landmark studies (see below) and do not consider HDL-C. Taking into account the most recent evidence and consensus statements, the author suggests the following approach:

1. All patients with type 2 diabetics or impaired glucose tolerance should be regarded as being at high risk and normally require aggressive correction of their adverse lipid profile.

2. The threshold for intervention should be the same as the target (see Chapter 4) for any of the following lipid parameters, with appropriate effective treatment to achieve and maintain values within the target range:
   - TC equal to or greater than 5.0mmol/l
   - LDL-C equal to or greater than 2.6 mmol/l
   - HDL-C equal to or less than 1.1 mmol/l
   - TG equal to or greater than 1.7 mmol/l

3. Irrespective of the baseline levels, improving the lipid profile will reduce cardiovascular risk in all type 2 diabetics, as supported by the studies cited below.

Non-pharmacological management of dyslipidaemia

The mainstay of non-pharmacological management is an improvement of lifestyle: dietary modification and increased physical activity, which are discussed elsewhere in this chapter. Weight loss, reduced alcohol intake and increased levels of physical activity can lead to decreased TG and LDL-C, and increased HDL-C levels. Improved glycaemic control can decrease TG levels. "Maximal" dietary modification can reduce LDL-C by up to 0.65 mmol/l.

Unless the patient is at high risk requiring immediate drug treatment, a period of from 3 to 6 months is needed to ascertain if the dietary and/or exercise regime has been successful.

Pharmacological management of dyslipidaemia

There are several classes of lipid-regulating drugs currently available (see the latest issues of BNF section 2.12 or of MIMS section 2H for doses). The statins (see below) have been regarded as the mainstay of lipid-regulating pharmacotherapy, but this drug class' main effect is to lower LDL-C without much improvement of either HDL-C or TG, both of which may be important. Therefore, prescribers will need to know about the other drug classes.

Ultimately, a combination of lipid-regulating drugs may need to be prescribed in high-risk individuals who require aggressive correction of their dyslipidaemia.

Anion-exchange resins (bile acid sequestrants)

The two available agents in this group of drugs are cholestyramine and colestipol. They act by binding bile acids in the gut, preventing their re-absorption. This promotes conversion of cholesterol into bile acids by the liver, resulting in increased LDL-receptor activity of hepatic cells which increases LDL-C clearance. In addition, since bile acids are required for the intestinal absorption of sterols, use of these agents results in increased faecal loss of dietary cholesterol. Although these drugs reduce LDL-C by up to 25% more than by dietary modification alone, they can aggravate hypertriglyceridaemia.

Anion-exchange resins are not especially palatable. They are not absorbed and can cause gastrointestinal side effects (constipation more than diarrhoea, nausea, vomiting and discomfort) and can interfere with the absorption of fat-soluble vitamins (A, D and K-supplementation may be necessary on long term therapy).

Fibrates

Fibrates (bezafibrate, ciprofibrate, fenofibrate and gemfibrozil) are broad spectrum lipid-modulating agents whose actions include:
- Decreased serum TG levels
- A reduction of LDL-C by up to 18%
- Increased HDL-C levels
- Decreased VLDL levels.

All fibrates can cause rhabdomyolysis or other muscle toxicities. These usually present as muscle pain, associated with elevated serum creatine phosphokinase (CPK), particularly in patients with impaired renal function or hypothyroidism. The risk of muscle toxicity is increased if a fibrate is taken concurrently with a statin or ciclosporin. Therefore, in patients taking a fibrate, CPK levels should be checked regularly and any muscle pains should be reported.

Bezafibrate suppresses endogenous synthesis of cholesterol and triglycerides. It also "causes the expression" of an increased number of specific LDL receptors, increasing the catabolism of LDL-C. Triglyceride catabolism is stimulated through systemic lipoprotein lipase and hepatic lipase. Ciprofibrate and fenofibrate lower plasma LDL, VLDL and TG levels and raise serum HDL levels without increasing the risk of developing gall stones. Gemfibrozil reduces raised levels of TG, TC, LDL-C and VLDL and raises low levels of HDL-C. Its lowering of plasma TG levels is likely to be achieved by reducing the hepatic synthesis of VLDL and increasing VLDL clearance.

Several studies provided good data to suggest that fibrates reduce CHD, although the extent of the effectiveness did vary. However, questions over safety were raised in two primary prevention studies[45,46], while two secondary prevention studies suggested that fibrates were quite safe[47,48].

It is hoped that the Fenofibrate Intervention and Event Lowering in Diabetes (FIELD) trial, due to report at the end of 2005, will provide the necessary evidence to clarify the precise role of fibrates in preventing CVD in patients with diabetes[49].

Statins (see below) are less effective in raising low HDL-C, recognised as being necessary in many patients with diabetes; therefore, alternative drug classes (such as fibrates and nicotinic acid group) are likely to be prescribed increasingly in lipid management. Despite the problems associated with combining gemfibrozil and the withdrawn statin cerivastatin, the need to raise HDL-C levels along with lowering LDL-C and TG levels may prompt the clinician to consider prescribing a statin-fibrate combination. More recent experience suggests that this combination is relatively safe, provided that renal, hepatic and thyroid function remains normal with CPK levels being monitored and that any muscle pains are promptly reported.

Statins

Hydroxymethyl glutaryl coenzyme A (HMG-CoA) reductase inhibitors are commonly known as statins and have been available for at least fifteen years. By competitive inhibition of the rate-limiting enzyme responsible for the hepatic synthesis of cholesterol, statins block the endogenous synthesis of cholesterol, causing the hepatocyte's cholesterol requirements to be met by the uptake of circulating cholesterol via a catabolic LDL receptor on the cell surface; the number of these receptors is thought to be increased by statins. Statins can reduce plasma LDL-C by up to 40%. These drugs also have a moderate effect on increasing HDL-C and lowering plasma TG levels, although this is less than their effect on LDL-C.

There are five statins currently available in the UK: atorvastatin, fluvastatin, pravastatin, rosuvastatin and simvastatin. Another statin, cerivastatin, was withdrawn due to the risk of rhabdomyolysis when it was used in combination with gemfibrozil (a fibrate).

Several well publicised trials demonstrated that pravastatin (CARE, LIPID and WOS) and simvastatin (4S and MRC/BHF) reduced both total and LDL cholesterol levels and were effective in the primary and secondary prevention of coronary heart disease. However, three recent landmark studies have provided the strongest evidence base for the benefits of lipid-lowering in patients with type 2 diabetes:

- The MRC/BHF Heart Protection Study reported that a lowering of LDL-C by 30% (using simvastatin) reduced the risk of a major CHD event by 25%, independent of the diabetic patient's baseline LDL-cholesterol[50].

- In 2004 the Collaborative AtoRvastatin Diabetes Study (CARDS) recruited 2,838 people with type 2 diabetes. It reported that there was a 37% reduction in the risk of a major coronary event in the group receiving atorvastatin 10mg compared with placebo. Acute coronary events were reduced by 36%, coronary revascularisation by 31% and stroke by 48% in the atorvastatin group. Baseline lipids, sex and age did not affect the results[51].

- The ASCOT primary prevention trial of high risk uncontrolled hypertensive patients recruited 2,532 patients with diabetes. In the lipid-lowering arm, subjects had a baseline non-fasting TC below 6.5mmol/l. The primary endpoint of non-fatal MI plus fatal CHD was reduced by over one third more in patients treated with atorvastatin 10mg compared to placebo, even with equivalent blood pressure reduction[52].

There is relatively little data available at present on the benefits of lipid-lowering therapy in patients with type 1 diabetes.

Although statins are usually well tolerated, they should be used with caution in patients with a history of liver disease or with a high alcohol intake. As with fibrates, rhabdomyolysis and reversible myositis are rare but significant side effects of statins, particularly in patients with renal impairment, hypothyroidism or taking concurrent fibrates or ciclosporin. CPK levels should be checked regularly and patients should be advised to report promptly unexplained muscle pain, tenderness or weakness.

Some patients treated with statins do not achieve their lipid-lowering goals. Drug combinations or alternatives need to be considered in these circumstances.

A "new generation" statin, rosuvastatin, is claimed by its manufacturers to be more potent at lowering LDL-C levels. This and other "superstatins" may become the subject of a NICE technology appraisal, due to concerns about their costs and the need to ascertain their precise role in lipid-lowering in comparison to the "older" statins.
In June 2004, revised guidance was issued for the prescribing of rosuvastatin, following reports to the U.S. Food and Drug Administration (FDA) and other regulatory bodies. There is an increased risk of serious muscle toxicity (myopathy), particularly in certain subpopulations (renal impairment, hypothyroidism, Japanese and Chinese origin, alcohol abuse, concomitant use of fibrates). It is advised that primary care should be prescribing mainly the lower doses of 5 to 10mg, with the maximum dose of 40mg to be prescribed only with greater caution and under close supervision.

Azetidinones
This drug group selectively inhibits cholesterol transport across the wall of the small intestine: thus, reducing the delivery of intestinal cholesterol to the liver. Ezetimibe is the first available product in this class. It is metabolised in the liver and small intestine to its active glucuronide form, which undergoes enterohepatic recycling, prolonging its action. Ezetimibe is not a bile acid sequestrant. It does not interfere with the absorption of TG, fatty acids or fat-soluble vitamins.

Ezetimibe's licenses include:
- Adjunctive therapy to dietary modification in patients with hypercholesterolaemia, either in combination with a statin (acting synergistically to lower LDL-C levels) or as monotherapy (if a statin is inappropriate or contra-indicated).
- Treatment of homozygous familial hypercholesterolaemia in combination with dietary modification and a statin.

Headache, abdominal pain and diarrhoea are common side effects of ezetimibe. Its effect on CVD morbidity and mortality is unknown. Adding ezetimibe to a statin is no safer and much more expensive than maximising the dosage of the statin[53]. However, where aggressive LDL-C lowering is required, ezetimibe may have a role: either in combination with a statin beyond a maximal statin dose or as an alternative if statins are contra-indicated or not tolerated.

Nicotinic acid group
The nicotinic acid group (nicotinic acid and acipimox are currently available) of drugs improve both serum cholesterol and triglyceride levels.

They appear to act in several ways, including partial inhibition of free fatty acid release from adipose tissue, increased lipoprotein lipase activity and decreased hepatic synthesis of LDL-C; thus producing lower LDL-C and triglyceride levels. Nicotinic acid can also increase HDL-C levels. Nicotinic acid's side effects, especially vasodilatation, can be troublesome.

Nicotinic acid is now available also in an extended-release formulation (Niaspan), which is currently more widely prescribed in the US than in the UK. Patients started on niaspan may experience transient facial flushing. This drug has been associated with hepatic toxicity; thus, liver function should be monitored prior and during prescribing. Niaspan should be used with caution in patients with a history of liver disease or who consume large quantities of alcohol.

In April 2004 the Scottish Medicines Consortium advised that Niaspan was not recommended for the treatment of hypercholesterolaemia and mixed hyperlipidaemia, due to the lack of suitable studies (available at the time) comparing it with other lipid-regulating drugs. However, as with fibrates, the need for aggressive lipid-regulation (especially if seeking to raise HDL-C levels and lower TG levels) may prompt clinicians to consider prescribing nicotinic acid, particularly in combination with a statin, subject to the cautions stated above.

Acipimox has fewer side effects than nicotinic acid, but may be less effective.

Fish oils

Fish oils reduce serum triglycerides. There are two preparations currently available:

1. Omega-3-acid ethyl esters (Omacor).

2. Omega-3 marine triglycerides (Maxepa). This can sometimes aggravate hypercholesterolaemia.

In the current climate of a more aggressive approach to lipid-regulation, this group of drugs is likely to be scrutinised more closely in the future.

Other drug groups

Other pharmacological options include:

- plant sterols (no drug preparation, not especially effective), and

- antioxidants (lack of supporting evidence from intervention studies).

Promising cholesterol management agents in development include:

1. Avasimibe, an acyl coenzyme A cholesterol acyltransferase (ACAT) inhibitor. It is a direct-acting anti-atherosclerotic agent and is in Phase III trials.

2. A cholesteryl ester transfer protein (CETP) inhibitor (JTT-705). This acts by increasing HDL-C levels and is in Phase II trials.

3. A cholesterol vaccine against endogenous CETP. This may be useful in reducing atherosclerosis risk factors. It, too, is in Phase II trials.

As Table 5.11 shows, the choice of drug prescribed depends upon the nature of the dyslipidaemia (not all patients need a statin), and the usual care over tolerability, contra-indications and potential interactions.

Once started on treatment, patients require earlier review to monitor the response to and the safety of their treatment. Patients on statins should have liver function test (LFTs) and creatine kinase (CK) estimations two to three months after starting treatment, after a further increase in dose, or if symptoms of myositis occur at any time on therapy.

Table 5.10: *Summary of the National Clinical Guideline's 2002 Recommendations for lipid lowering pharmacological therapy in patients with type 2 diabetes*

Blood lipid profile at the start of therapy (mmol/l)	10-year coronary event risk	Recommendations
TC ≥ 5.0 or LDL-C ≥ 3.0 or TG ≥ 2.3, but ≤ 10	Lower: No history of CVD **and** 10-year coronary event risk ≤ 15%	• Discuss CHD risk, considering treatment options • Consider offering drug therapy at higher TC & TG levels • If decided to start treatment, offer statin • Monitor treatment 3 monthly and titrate until stable • If decision made not to prescribe drugs, monitor lipid profile annually
TC ≥ 5.0 or LDL-C ≥ 3.0 or TG ≥ 2.3, but ≤ 10	Higher: 10-year coronary event risk ≥ 15%, **but** no CVD history	**Primary prevention** • Offer a statin • Monitor treatment 3 monthly and titrate until stable • Monitor lipid profile annually
TC ≥ 5.0 or LDL-C ≥ 3.0 or TG ≥ 2.3, but ≤ 10	**Higher:** manifest CVD	**Secondary prevention** • Offer a statin • Monitor treatment in 3 months and titrate • Consider adding fibrate after 6 months if TG remains ≥ 2.3 • Monitor for interaction between statin & fibrate • Monitor lipid profile annually
TC < 5.0 *or* LDL-C < 3.0 **and** TG ≥ 2.3, but ≤10	**Higher:** manifest CVD	**Secondary prevention** • Offer a statin or a fibrate • Monitor treatment 3 monthly and titrate until stable • Monitor lipid profile annually
Fasting TG > 10	**Higher or lower**	• Offer fibrate therapy • Consider referral to specialist clinic

Key:
TC = total cholesterol   TG = triglycerides   CHD = coronary heart disease   CVD = cardiovascular disease

The author has slightly modified the very good summary from the American Diabetes Association (see Table 5.11) of the appropriate therapeutic interventions for the different types of dyslipidaemia in patients with diabetes.

Table 5.11: Order of priorities for treatment of diabetic dyslipidaemia[54]

Main treatment aim	1st Choice	2nd Choice	3rd Choice
LDL cholesterol lowering	Statin	Anion-exchange resin OR Fibrate	
HDL cholesterol raising	Behavioural: 1. Weight loss 2. Increased exercise 3. Smoking cessation	Behavioural PLUS Fibrate OR Nicotinic acid	
Triglyceride lowering	Optimal glycaemic control	Fibrate	Statin at high dose (especially if raised LDL)
Combined hyperlipidaemia	Optimal glycaemic control PLUS Statin	Optimal glycaemic control PLUS Statin PLUS Fibrate*	Optimal glycaemic control PLUS Statin PLUS Nicotinic acid

*The combination of a statin with nicotinic acid or, especially a fibrate, may increase the risk of myositis: monitor hepatic, renal and thyroid function, as well as CPK.

Recently published landmark studies (MRF/BHF, ASCOT and CARDS) do suggest that, for dyslipidaemia in patients with diabetes (especially type 2), not only may the targets for treatment (see Chapter 4) need to change, but also the choice of therapeutic interventions. It is possible that the accepted therapeutic approach will become "statins for all patients with type 2 diabetes", with the other drug groups being used only if statins are not tolerated or if combination therapy is needed to produce a greater change in the lipid profile. In patients with type 2 diabetes and hypertension, routine use of a statin (irrespective of baseline LDL-cholesterol) is now being recommended by the BHS[25], although the benefits of lipid-lowering in the elderly has not been established.

A note of caution needs to be introduced at this point. Statins do not produce significant increases in low HDL-C levels. Also, women and non-Caucasians were not always well represented in lipid-lowering interventional studies and there are no published studies reporting the effect of lipid-lowering therapy on "hard" cardiovascular outcomes in any population originating from the Indian subcontinent[55]. As discussed in Chapter 2, being a female and/or non-white diabetic does increase an individual's susceptibility to the adverse effects of many cardiovascular risk factors. However, it is reasonable for the time-being, until further evidence is published, not to allow the patient's gender or ethnicity to influence decisions about the type of therapy to reduce cardiovascular risk.

Referral to either a lipid clinic or a diabetic clinic is indicated if there is failure to achieve the targets or if the medication used causes problems.

Optimising glycaemic control

Other resources provide more detailed guidance about optimising glycaemic control (see Appendix 4). As discussed in Chapter 2, chronic hyperglycaemia is associated with increased cardiovascular risk, although this association may be weaker than for smoking, dyslipidaemia and hypertension. The evidence base for improved glycaemic control reducing cardiovascular events is still not overwhelmingly strong. However, chronic hyperglycaemia does have a closer association with microvascular diabetic complications, and better glycaemic control has been shown to reduce the risk of these adverse outcomes occurring.

Optimal glycaemic control is a balance between three components: diet, physical activity, and blood glucose-lowering medication. Diet and physical activity are discussed elsewhere in this chapter.

The blood glucose-lowering medication for patients with type 1 diabetes is insulin; whereas blood glucose in patients with type 2 diabetes can be treated with diet alone, oral medication or insulin, with the latter two being combined in some individuals.

Oral drug therapy

Overview
In patients with type 2 diabetes there is likely to be a progressive deterioration over time of pancreatic ß-cell function, resulting in most patients eventually requiring insulin to achieve acceptable glycaemic control. The main classes of oral blood glucose lowering medication act by improving either insulin secretion or insulin action. In order for a drug

to stimulate insulin secretion, it is necessary that the pancreatic ß-cells are still functioning. Further details about the drug classes discussed below can be found in the BNF (section 6.1.2).

The author has found useful a stepped approach to altering blood glucose-lowering treatment in patients with type 2 diabetes, starting with diet alone or monotherapy and moving onto logical and effective combinations of different agents. This approach is summarised in Table 5.12, with more than one option at some numbered steps, the choice depending upon the patient's circumstances.

The combination of self-monitoring results, a recent HbA1c result, and the patient's well-being should guide both dose changes and decisions about additional medication (or a step-up). The interval between any dose changes must allow sufficient time for their effect to be seen, but prompt action is indicated in the event of repeated hypoglycaemia or significant hyperglycaemia. Ideally, additional medication should be introduced only after the maximum recommended dose of current medication has failed to achieve reasonable glycaemic control or is not tolerated. A patient's concordance with treatment needs to be discussed and monitored where glycaemic control appears problematic.

Notwithstanding the benefits and need for the various drugs described below in achieving and maintaining good glycaemic control, the one agent that has been shown most clearly to reduce mortality is metformin (see below), an inexpensive drug that has been available for many years.

Oral drug therapy that improves insulin secretion (insulin secretagogues)

Despite considerable pharmacokinetic differences, the two main groups of insulin secretagogues (sulphonylureas and postprandial glucose regulators) both act by closing the potassium channel of the islet ß-cell, thus promoting membrane depolarisation, calcium influx and insulin granule release into the extracellular medium. Therefore, all of these drugs require that some residual pancreatic ß-cell activity is present. They do not affect insulin resistance.

Sulphonylureas and postprandial glucose regulators are alternatives to each other and not meant to be used in combination. Because all of these drugs promote insulin secretion, they should be taken prior to meals for ideal effect.

There is considerable evidence that insulin secretagogues are effective in reducing blood glucose levels. In the UKPDS, sulphonylureas are among the therapies that were shown to reduce vascular complications, when compared to lifestyle interventions alone.

Table 5.12: *Summary of the treatment of raised blood glucose in type 2 diabetes*[56]

Step	Evaluation	Intervention
1	a. Ketonuria absent b. Fasting blood glucose is <15 mmol/l	Dietary advice
2a	a. Ketonuria absent b. Fasting blood glucose is ≥15 mmol/l OR failure of diet to control blood glucose c. Obese (BMI >25 kg/m²) d. Absence of renal (creatinine >130nmol/l), hepatic or cardiac impairment OR risk of sudden deterioration	Metformin (Thiazolidinedione as alternative in renal impairment or if intolerant of metformin)
2b	As in 2a, but non-obese or intolerant of metformin	Insulin secretagogue [Sulphonylurea OR PPRG* (if irregular meals)]
3a	a. Ketonuria absent b. Failure of first-line drug to control blood glucose c. Absence of renal, hepatic or cardiac impairment	**Combination** of Metformin AND Insulin secretagogue
3b	a. Ketonuria absent b. Failure of metformin and sulphonylurea combination to control blood glucose c. Absence of renal, hepatic or cardiac impairment d. Intolerance of either 1st line drug e. Obese	**Combination** of Thiazolidinedione AND Metformin (preferable, especially if obese) OR Sulphonylurea
4	a. Ketonuria absent b. Failure of double therapy c. Absence of renal, hepatic or cardiac impairment d. Very obese OR unwilling to consider insulin therapy	**Combination** of Rosiglitazone, Metformin AND Sulphonylurea
5	Failure to control blood glucose with oral agents	Insulin WITH OR WITHOUT Metformin (in the absence of renal, hepatic or cardiac impairment) OR Sulphonylurea

*Repaglinide (meglitinide) can be prescribed either as monotherapy or in combination with metformin, but nateglinide is currently licensed only in combination with metformin.

NICE's Clinical Guidelines in 2002[57] recommended that:
- Insulin secretagogues should be used in combination with metformin in overweight people when adequate glycaemic control had not been achieved.
- Insulin secretagogues should be considered as a first line option in people not overweight or in whom metformin is contra-indicated or not tolerated.
- A generic sulphonylurea should "normally" be the insulin secretagogue of choice.

Sulphonylureas

This class of drugs is long-established, with the following agents available (more details in Appendix 1): tolbutamide, glibenclamide (glyburide), gliclazide (also available in a modified-release formulation), glimepiride, gliquidone, glipizide and chlorpropamide. Chlorpropamide has more side-effects and drawbacks than the other sulphonylureas and is no longer recommended. Choice needs to take account of side-effects and duration of action, as well as the patient's age and renal function; the different sulphonylureas appear to have a comparable effect upon blood glucose-lowering. Sulphonylureas can be combined with either metformin, a glitazone, basal insulin or acarbose.

Although both once-daily and twice-daily dosing are associated with better concordance (see Chapter 4), once-daily preparations have the advantages of reducing the total number of tablets that a patient needs to take and of often simplifying the drug regimen.

Sulphonylureas are contra-indicated in severe hepatic and renal impairment, porphyria, during breast-feeding and pregnancy, and when ketoacidosis is present. The short-acting tolbutamide can be used in renal impairment, as can gliclazide and gliquidone, which are metabolised mainly in the liver. The side-effects of sulphonylureas are mild and infrequent, and include gastro-intestinal disturbances and hypersensitivity reactions (a skin rash that usually appears within 6 to 8 weeks of initiation).

The two drawbacks associated with sulphonylureas have been that they can induce hypoglycaemia and can encourage weight gain (see BNF 6.1.2.1 cautions). These were found in the long-acting drugs, chlorpropamide and glibenclamide. Glibenclamide is associated with the rare but potentially fatal occurrence of nocturnal hypoglycaemia in the elderly. Weight gain was recorded with both chlorpropamide and glibenclamide (but less than with insulin) in the intensively treated group of patients in the UKPDS[58].

However, hypoglycaemia and weight gain are not inevitable with this drug class, and the risks of either occurring may be minimised by:
- Avoiding the long-acting agents, chlorpropamide and glibenclamide.
- Avoiding use in patients with mild to moderate hepatic and renal impairment, and being careful about use in the elderly.

- Careful introduction and dose titration of the drug (according to the results of self-monitoring).
- Using the lowest dose that achieves and maintains normoglycaemia.

Postprandial regulators of glucose (PPRG)

These drugs increase early (first phase) insulin secretion in response to rising plasma glucose levels by pancreatic beta cells, reducing the mealtime "glucose spike". In contrast, sulphonylureas have less effect on this first phase. The two available drugs in this group are repaglinide and nateglinide. Both can be used in combination with metformin, but nateglinide is not currently licensed for monotherapy.

PPRGs have a quick onset and a short duration of action. They are best initiated at an earlier stage in the disease process when pancreatic β-cells still have a reasonable capacity to secrete insulin. PPRGs may be preferred to sulphonylureas in a type 2 diabetic who either needs to fast (e.g. a Muslim during Ramadan) or whose meal times are unpredictable and/or irregular.

PPRGs should be avoided in patients with severe liver disease or on dialysis, and in pregnancy, breastfeeding and ketoacidosis. The potential side-effects of both drugs include hypoglycaemia and hypersensitivity reactions, and repaglinide can be associated with gastro-intestinal disturbances.

Oral drug therapy that improves insulin action (by reducing insulin resistance)

Biguanides

Metformin is the only available drug in this class. It is the first choice drug for obese type 2 patients, but it is an option for first-line therapy in the non-obese. It works by decreasing gluconeogenesis in the liver and by increasing glucose uptake in peripheral tissues.

Metformin can be combined with all other blood glucose-lowering drug groups. In the UKPDS study treatment with metformin was shown to reduce all-cause mortality by 36% in comparison to treatment with either insulin or a sulphonylurea[59].

Its main side effects are on the gastro-intestinal tract, lessened by a stepped approach to increasing the dose and by its being taken with or after food. There is a slight risk of precipitating lactic acidosis with metformin in vulnerable individuals. Therefore, it should not be used in the presence of renal (creatinine greater than 130nmol/l), hepatic or cardiac impairment (particularly if the patient is being treated with a β-blocker), tissue hypoxia (e.g. sepsis, respiratory failure, recent myocardial infarction) and concurrent use of iodine-containing X-ray contrast media (do not restart metformin until renal function returns to normal). Metformin should be avoided in type 2 diabetics with alcohol problems. Some experts recommend regular serum creatinine and B12 estimations in patients on long-term metformin.

Thiazolidinediones – also known as glitazones[60]

These drugs act by promoting glucose utilisation peripherally, which enhances insulin action, but does not affect insulin secretion. They are thought to activate receptors, located mainly in adipose tissue, that affect glucose and lipid metabolism and to maintain insulin secretion in pancreatic beta cells[61] by reducing the effect of glucose "toxicity". Two agents, rosiglitazone and pioglitazone, were launched in the UK in 2000.

These agents can be prescribed as monotherapy, in combination with either metformin OR a sulphonylurea, or in triple therapy with metformin AND a sulphonylurea (rosiglitazone only, as pioglitazone is not currently licenced for triple therapy). Their current UK licence does not include prescribing in combination with PPRG or insulin. The combination of a glitazone and metformin is logical if reducing insulin resistance is the main aim of therapy.

In August 2003, NICE recommended their use mainly in those unable to take metformin and a sulphonylurea in combination because of lack of tolerance or a contraindication to one of these drugs[62]. In the following month, the European Medicines Agency (EMEA) extended the license of glitazones to allow monotherapy.[63] In 2004, the Association of British Clinical Diabetologists (ABCD) produced a position statement that included the following recommendations for patients with type 2 diabetes[64]:

- A glitazone is the preferred second-line oral agent in addition to metformin in the obese.

- A glitazone can replace metformin in renal impairment.

- A glitazone is not a substitute for insulin if poor control on maximal tolerated metformin and sulphonylurea combination.

- Triple therapy, with rosiglitazone, metformin and a sulphonylurea, may be considered in the very obese or in patients unwilling to go onto insulin.

- Glitazones should not be used in combination with insulin, in heart failure, or in patients with pre-treatment serum transaminase levels more than 2.5 times the upper limit of normal.

When prescribing a glitazone, liver function needs to be monitored. Both glitazones can cause weight gain, in part due to fluid retention that may precipitate heart failure, particularly if the glitazone is combined with insulin.

Short-term data suggests that both glitazones may have some blood pressure lowering effect. The effects that both glitazones have on lipid parameters are mixed. Further short-term data from pioglitazone's manufacturers shows that both drugs appear to demonstrate equivalent improved glycaemic control, but increase both HDL-C (good news) and LDL-C (bad news), although it was suggested that the changes to the lipid profile were significantly more favourable with pioglitazone[65].

As this book goes to press, there are several ongoing randomised controlled clinical trials to assess what effect glitazones may have upon cardiovascular risk and outcomes. Both metformin and sulphonylureas reduce vascular complications. Do glitazones have similar or comparable benefits? Table 5.13 summarises some studies that should, hopefully, provide the answer.

Table 5.13: Summary of ongoing RCTs of glitazones' effects upon cardiovascular outcomes in patients with type 2 diabetes[66]

Study	Description	Outcome	Subjects	Completetion date and duration
PROactive	Pioglitazone vs. placebo	Total mortality, macrovascular morbidity	5,238 high cardiovascular risk	2005 (4 years)
ADOPT	Rosiglitazone vs. metformin vs. glibenclamide	Disease progression, ß-cell function, risk markers for macrovascular complications	4,356 drug-naïve	2006 (4-6 years)
RECORD	Rosiglitazone plus metformin or sulphonylurea vs. metformin plus sulphonylurea	Cardiovascular outcomes	3,966 inadequately controlled on either metformin or sulphonylurea	2009 (6 years)

Table 5.14: *Overview of insulin preparations*[67]

Category	Generic types	Proprietary examples	Onset of action (minutes)	Peak of action (hours)	Duration of action
Rapid-acting	Lispro, Aspart	Humalog, NovoRapid	15 15	$1/4$ to 2 $1/2$ to 3	4 5
Short-acting	Regular	Actrapid, Velosulin Hypurin, Humulin S, Insuman Rapid	15 – 60	1 – 6	4 – 12
Rapid-acting and intermediate-acting	Biphasic insulin aspart, Biphasic insulin lispro	NovoMix30, HumalogMix 25 or 50	10 - 20	2 peaks (as for its components)	12 - 18
Short-acting and intermediate-acting (Biphasic)	Regular – isophane (NPH) mixture	Mixtard 10-50, Humulin M3, Hypurin 30, InsumanComb 15, 25, 50	15 – 60	2 peaks (as for its components)	12 – 18
Intermediate-acting (Basal)	Isophane (NPH)	Insulatard, Hypurin, Humulin I, Insuman Basal	60 – 120	4 – 8	12 – 18
Long-acting	Crystalline zinc suspensions (insulin zinc suspension)	Monotard, Hypurin Lente, Ultratard	120 – 240	6 – 18	18 – >24
Newer	Insulin glargine	Lantus	150	Plateau	23

Other oral drugs

Another drug currently available in the UK is acarbose (Glucobay). It inhibits intestinal alpha-glucosidase, delaying the digestion of starch and sucrose that increase blood glucose levels following ingestion of carbohydrate. The result is a fall in post-prandial glucose and insulin levels. Acarbose can be prescribed either as monotherapy or in combination with other oral agents. It does not cause weight gain and is unlikely to cause hypoglycaemia as monotherapy. Unfortunately, its widespread use is limited by its gastrointestinal side effects (occurring in up to 60% of patients). These are dose dependent, and include flatulence, bloating and diarrhoea.

Insulin

Insulin Preparations

There is a wide variety of insulin preparations now available. Insulins can be classified according to their onset and duration of action, shown in Table 5.14. Insulins also vary according to their origin and method of manufacture (animal-derived, semi-synthetic or synthetic), modifications which alter duration of action, and their mode of delivery (e.g. syringe, pen, infusion device – see below).

Onset and duration of action

Different pharmaceutical companies have adopted different names for the same insulins or their mixtures. Further details are available in the latest issues of the BNF (Section 6.1.1) or MIMS (Section 7A).

1. Rapid-acting insulins:

These recently developed insulins have both a more rapid onset and shorter duration of action than the "short-acting insulins. Further details are in the subsection below on modifications to insulin.

2. Short-acting insulins:

There are many preparations now available. Ideally, short-acting insulin should be given 30 to 45 minutes before meals to match its peak action to glucose absorption from the gastrointestinal tract. A delayed meal risks hypoglycaemia and injecting just before, during or after a meal will not facilitate tight glycaemic control, as the insulin's onset of action may occur after it is most needed. In these circumstances, rapid-acting insulin may be more effective.

3. Intermediate-acting insulins:

The long-established isophane preparations, also known as neutral protamine Hagedorn (NPH), are produced by complexing insulin with protamine. Although they can be used as monotherapy either once or twice daily, they are often mixed with either rapid- or short-acting insulins. They can also be given as a single bedtime dose, combined with daytime oral agents in patients with type 2 diabetes (see below). For convenience, premixed insulins (also known as biphasic) are available, containing both short- or rapid-acting and intermediate-acting insulins (e.g. Mixtard, Humulin M, and Humalog Mix) in various proportions. In European nomenclature the short-acting percentage is given in the preparation's proprietary name. The 30% mixture is often favoured in the UK.

4. Long-acting insulins:

These are becoming less popular, because their mixture with shorting-acting insulins causes problems, and because premixed and prolonged-acting analogue insulins have now become available and are being increasingly used in preference.

Origin and method of manufacture

Short-, intermediate- and long-acting insulins are either based on the human sequence of amino acids or are extracted from an animal pancreas, usually porcine (less antigenic than beef), and then purified. Synthetic human insulin is produced either by enzyme modification of porcine insulin (emp) or, more commonly, from a proinsulin synthesised by bacteria (prb) or from a precursor synthesised by yeast (pyr), both using recombinant DNA technology. Human insulins have a more rapid onset of action and a shorter duration of activity than porcine insulins[67].

Modifications which alter the onset and duration of action

Recently, insulin analogues have been introduced that are genetically engineered, containing modifications to soluble human insulin. These include:

- **Rapid-acting**, e.g. lispro (transposes two amino acids, lysine and praline, on the B chain to B28 lysine and B29 proline) and aspart (aspartate replaces praline at B28). These have a rapid onset and a short duration of action.

- **Prolonged-acting**. There are currently two basal insulin analogues available in the UK. Both have a prolonged plateau of concentration rather than a peak (less risk of hypoglycaemia); and both have a duration of activity just under 24 hours; a once daily injection can often cover a patient's daily basal insulin needs. Because of these features, the new analogues may well replace isophane as the basal insulin of choice.

1. Insulin glargine (two additional arginine molecules are placed at B31 and B32, at the C terminus of the B chain, and arginine replaces asparagines at A21- the latter makes the molecule more stable). Insulin glargine should be administered in the evening or at bedtime. When converting to insulin glargine from isophane, the dosage should be 20% less than the total 24 hour dose of the previous basal insulin.

2. Insulin detemir (Levemir) was launched in the UK in 2004. It is administered once or twice daily. When converting to insulin detemir from isophane, the total dosage does not require adjustment if the pre-meal blood glucose averages 6.5 mmol/l or less; however, the total dosage should be increased by 10%, 20% and 25% if the pre-meal blood glucose averages, respectively, 6.6 to 10 mmol/l, 10.1 to 15 mmol/l and >15 mmol/l. When both pre-breakfast and pre-dinner targets cannot be reached, then consider splitting the total daily insulin detemir dose into two injections.

Both basal insulin analogues can used either on their own or in combination with oral agents (metformin or sulphonylurea), or with short- or rapid-acting insulin (see below for details of possible regimens).

Possible insulin regimens

The insulin regimen used has to be tailored to the patient's needs and lifestyle, and it must take into account the patient's wishes and sensitivities. Rapid-, short-, intermediate-, and long-acting insulin preparations may be injected either separately or mixed together in the same syringe.

Four regimens are available; the first two are suitable for both type 1 and type 2 diabetes, but the third and fourth can only be used in patients with type 2 diabetes:

1. The most popular regimen is to give **twice daily insulin before meals in the morning and evening**. The basis of this regimen is intermediate-acting insulin (often two thirds of the total daily dose is given before breakfast and one third before the evening meal or at bedtime); however, this is often given in combination with a rapid- or short-acting insulin, either drawn up separately or as a pre-mixed combination.

2. The basal bolus regimen: **Rapid-acting insulin three times daily** before breakfast, midday and evening meal, with either **twice daily intermediate-acting or a single injection of prolonged acting insulin (e.g. insulin glargine) at bedtime**. If using Humalog Mix (rapid- and intermediate-acting insulin mixture) twice daily, it is still possible to give an additional dose of rapid-acting insulin in-between to cover a large meal.

3. **Once daily insulin** (with basal insulin, such as intermediate-acting isophane) may be appropriate for those patients (e.g. a frail, isolated elderly diabetic) in whom tight blood glucose control is not the main therapeutic goal or where hypoglycaemia may be disastrous. Insulin glargine or insulin detemir may prove more useful alternatives.

4. **Combination of an intermediate-acting or prolonged-acting insulin once daily at bedtime AND oral hypoglycaemic drug(s) during the day** (e.g. a sulphonylurea), when the oral combination of a hypoglycaemic drug (other than metformin) with a sulphonylurea has failed to achieve satisfactory glycaemic control. This regimen has not been shown to be more effective than insulin alone, but the combination may be more practical for some patients.

In patients with type 2 diabetes it is possible to combine metformin with any of the above insulin regimens in order to overcome insulin resistance. There is good evidence that better glycaemic control, weight loss and reduced risk of hypoglycaemia are more likely when using a metformin and insulin combination.

Insulin dose adjustment

Insulin doses need to be titrated against blood glucose levels, aiming for 4 to 7 mmol/l before meals. It may take a few weeks to achieve normal blood glucose levels. Recurrent hypos, weight gain, wildly variable blood glucose values, and subtle features of chronic hypoglycaemia (headache, personality change in elderly, the need to eat) are suggestive of chronic over-dose of insulin.

There is no single set of advice to cope with every situation. However, there are a number of guiding principles that may help:

- Try to avoid changing insulin on the basis of a one-off reading

- Review also monitoring and injection techniques, eating and activity levels and patterns

- Consider distribution as well as quantity of insulin

- Look for patterns: identify periods of the day with greatest problems

- Agree finite dose changes, e.g. 2 units, and allow an interval of a few days between dose changes to allow the patient time to adapt and ascertain effect.

Reducing alcohol consumption

It is well beyond the scope of this book to discuss in great detail the treatment of excess alcohol consumption. Where the weekly consumption of alcohol is far above the recognised safe upper limit and/or there is resulting organ damage or characteristic deviant behaviour, the management may include in-patient admission for withdrawal or for the treatment of severe physical illness. Such situations require considerable resources and need to involve those with special interest and expertise in the field. However, at the centre of reducing alcohol consumption is the patient's willingness and commitment to change. The principles are the same as for patients who do not have diabetes.

Health professionals in primary care can play a very useful role in a variety of ways:

1. Evaluating willingness and barriers to change, and any target organ damage.

2. Support of withdrawal, supplementing the drug treatment with vitamins (especially thiamine), and being encouraging as appropriate.

3. Liaising with other services (such as the local alcohol team).

4. Supporting the patient's family where needed.

Behavioural change may still be required in patients whose alcohol consumption is excessive, but not resulting in severe physical, psychological and social problems.

Anti-platelet therapy

In addition to the risk factors discussed elsewhere in this book, platelets contribute to the development of atherosclerosis and vascular thrombosis. *In vitro* evidence suggests that patients with diabetes are often more sensitive to platelet-aggregating agents. Thromboxane is a potent vasoconstrictor and platelet aggregator. In patients with type 2 diabetes and cardiovascular disease, thromboxane production is increased. Aspirin blocks thromboxane synthesis by acetylating platelet cyclo-oxygenase.

Aspirin has a role in the primary and secondary prevention of cardiovascular events in patients without and with diabetes mellitus. There is considerable evidence from trials and meta-analyses that low-dose aspirin should be prescribed for secondary prevention, unless contra-indicated. Furthermore, the evidence also shows that low-dose aspirin (75 to 162mg/day) is equally effective and, possibly, less risky than at higher doses. Despite its proven efficacy, aspirin is under-prescribed in patients with diabetes[69].

The major risks of aspirin therapy are damage to the gastric mucosa and gastro-intestinal haemorrhage, even at relatively low doses. There is also an increased risk of minor bleeding episodes, such as epistaxis and bruising, but not retinal or vitreous haemorrhage. Enteric coated preparations do not appear to reduce this risk. The contra-indications to prescribing aspirin are allergy, bleeding tendency, concurrent anticoagulation treatment, recent gastro-intestinal haemorrhage, history of asthma triggered by asthma, uncontrolled hypertension, and clinically active hepatic disease.

Clopidogrel (75mg) may be considered as an alternative to aspirin in patients allergic to aspirin. It is also rather more expensive. There is limited data in patients with diabetes, but one large study found clopidogrel to be slightly more effective than 325mg aspirin in reducing the combined risk of stroke, myocardial infarction, or vascular death in a non-diabetic and diabetic study population[70]. Aspirin and clopidogrel are sometimes combined.

In order to minimise the risk of a cerebro-vascular event, it is recommended that aspirin is commenced only when blood pressure is controlled to less than 150/90. The latest guidance from the American Diabetes Association on aspirin therapy includes the following:

- Aspirin at a daily dose of 75–150mg daily should be used, unless contraindicated, as secondary prevention in people with diabetes (both types 1 and 2) and a previous history of myocardial infarction, vascular bypass procedure, stroke or transient ischaemic attack, peripheral vascular disease, claudication, and/or angina pectoris.

- Aspirin at a daily dose of 75–150mg daily should be used, unless contraindicated, as primary prevention in people with type 2 diabetes and increased cardiovascular risk, including those aged over 40 years with the presence of an additional cardiovascular risk factor (such as family history of CVD, hypertension, smoking, dyslipidaemia and albuminuria).

- There is less strong evidence that aspirin at a daily dose of 75–150mg daily should be used, subject to contra-indications, as primary prevention in people with type 1 diabetes and increased cardiovascular risk, including those aged over 40 years with the presence of an additional cardiovascular risk factor (such as family history of CVD, hypertension, smoker, dyslipidaemia and albuminuria).

- Aspirin should not be prescribed to individuals under the age of 21 years, because of the increased risk of Reye's syndrome associated with aspirin use in this population.

Diabetes UK posted in April 2001 its care recommendation for aspirin treatment in diabetes[71]. It recommends a dose of 75mg daily in patients aged over 30 years for secondary prevention, as above, and for primary prevention with the presence of one or more additional cardiovascular risk factors, as above, but also a BMI greater than 25 kg/m[2] or more, South Asian ethnicity, or the presence of diabetic retinopathy.

Microalbuminuria

There have been several hospital-based studies showing that early intervention with angiotensin converting enzyme (ACE) inhibitor drugs can delay or prevent the development of diabetic renal disease in types 1[72,73] and 2[74] patients, even when normotensive. Recent reports suggest that angiotensin-receptor antagonists (ARB) are reno-protective in type 2 diabetics with either hypertension and microalbuminuria or more overt nephropathy[75]. Further evidence is required to determine whether type 2 diabetics with particular characteristics (level of blood pressure, degree of nephropathy, ethnic group) would benefit from drugs that inhibit the renin-angiotensin-aldosterone system (with an ACE inhibitor or an ARB).

Although blockade of the renin-angiotensin system is the mainstay of treatment to delay the progression of microalbuminuria, smoking cessation and improved metabolic control should be included, as appropriate.

Reducing cardiovascular risk in patients with both diabetes and CHD

The precise efficacy of each intervention discussed above in reducing cardiovascular risk may vary depending upon the characteristics of the individual patient. Nevertheless, certain interventions, such as blood pressure-lowering, smoking cessation and improving lipid profiles will benefit virtually any patient with diabetes.

When a patient with diabetes is also known to have CHD, then a comprehensive and aggressive approach should be used to reduce further an already sizeable cardiovascular risk. Table 5.15 summarises the relevant interventions (subject to contra-indications and cautions) that have been shown to improve cardiovascular outcomes in patients with both diabetes and known CHD. Management involves combining all reasonable interventions of proven benefit.

Significantly reducing a patient's cardiovascular risk is often difficult, requires collaboration and is life-long, but the potential benefits for the patient may outweigh the associated adverse effects of treatment in the long-term. As stated earlier in this book, the risk of a CVD event occurring can be reduced or delayed, but never prevented totally. Ultimately, the health professional's job is to "tilt" the odds more in his patient's favour.

Table 5.15: Summary of interventions for secondary CHD prevention in patients with diabetes [76]

1. Blood pressure reduction
2. Smoking cessation
3. Aspirin 75 to 150mg daily (clopidogrel 75mg daily if aspirin intolerant)
4. Oral anticoagulation (if severe LV dysfunction post-MI, persistent AF and/or mural or left atrial thrombus), with target INR of 2 to 3.
5. Selective beta-1 blocker (avoid beta blocker with ISA)
6. ACE inhibition, especially if congestive heart failure and/or LV ejection fraction <35%; to prevent or slow the progression of nephropathy
7. Lower LDL-cholesterol < 2.0 mmol/l; increase HDL-cholesterol > 1.0 mmol/l
8. Optimal glycaemic control
9. Avoid calcium channel blockers, except if LV function is preserved and beta-blockers are contra-indicated
10. Optimal medical nutrition therapy
11. Increased suitable physical activity
12. Reduction of obesity

■ Key messages:

- Health education is central to enabling and supporting a patient in improving adverse health behaviour. Education is much more than imparting information; it involves altering motivation and supporting change.

- Interventions need to be tailored to the needs and circumstances of the individual patient.

- Modifying many risk factors requires a combination of interventions to be undertaken.

- Interventions for which there is evidence that cardiovascular outcomes are improved should be preferred to those which simply improve risk factors.

- Treatment of hypertension in patients with type 2 diabetes should normally be accompanied by use of a statin, irrespective of baseline lipid levels, unless elderly.

- For modifying some risk factors, the result of treatment is often more important than the theoretical advantages of selecting a particular therapy. Frequently, there is more than one way to achieve an improvement.

Appendix 1
Formulary of Medication Available in the UK

Further details are found in the latest editions of the British National Formulary (BNF) and the Monthly Index of Medical Specialities (MIMS). The author has based the cost calculations on data from the April 2005 issues of the Drug Tariff (for generic drugs) and MIMS (for proprietary drugs). The costs are to the NHS, excluding VAT. Readers should bear in mind that costs are constantly changing.

Smoking cessation products

Generic name	Proprietary name(s)	Daily dose range	NHS cost for 28 days (£)
Bupropion	Zyban	150mg for 6 days; then 150mg twice daily	37.19
Nicotine	Nicorette Nicotinell NiQuitin CQ	Depends upon preparation	various

Anti-obesity drugs

Generic name	Proprietary name(s)	Daily dose range	NHS cost for 28 days (£)	Comments (see NICE guidance)
Orlistat	Xenical	360mg in 3 doses after meals	39.51	Lipase inhibitor, reducing dietary fat absorption
Sibutramine	Reductil	10 to 15mg in 1 dose	41.29 – 45.14	Centrally acting appetite suppressant, inhibiting re-uptake of noradrenaline and serotonin

Blood pressure-lowering drugs

Angiotensin converting enzyme (ACE) inhibitors

Generic name	Proprietary name(s)	Daily dose range	NHS cost for 28 days (£)
Captopril	Capoten	12.5mg in 2 doses to 150mg in 3 doses	0.85 – 2.67 (generic) 4.91 – 28.60 (proprietary)
Cilazapril	Vasace	0.5 – 5mg	3.65 – 13.28
Enalapril maleate	Innovace	2.5 – 40mg in 1 to 2 doses	1.00 – 3.20 (generic) 5.35 – 25.02 (proprietary)
Fosinopril	Staril	10 – 40mg	11.20 – 24.18
Imidapril hydrochloride	Tanatril	2.5 – 20mg	2.83 – 7.67
Lisinopril	Carace Zestril	2.5 – 80mg	1.76 – 9.72 (generic) 6.26 – 43.88 (proprietary)
Moexipril hydrochloride	Perdix	3.75 – 30mg	3.78 – 17.40
Perindopril	Coversyl	2 – 8mg	10.95 (all strengths)
Quinapril	Accupro	2.5 – 80mg in 1-2 doses	4.30 – 19.50
Ramipril	Tritace	1.25 – 10mg	2.26 – 2.98 (generic - capsules) 5.30 – 14.24 (proprietary)
Trandolapril	Gopten Odrik	0.5 – 4mg	3.42 – 14.24

Angiotensin II receptor antagonists (ARB)

Generic name	Proprietary name(s)	Daily dose range	NHS cost for 28 days (£)
Candesartan cilexetil	Amias	8 – 32mg	9.89 – 16.13
Eprosartan	Teveten	300 – 800mg	11.63 – 31.54
Irbesartan	Aprovel	75 – 300mg	10.29 – 16.91
Losartan potassium	Cozaar	25 –100mg	18.12 – 24.20
Olmesartan medoxomil	Olmetec	10 – 40mg	10.95 – 17.50
Telmisartan	Micardis	20 – 80mg	11.34 – 14.18
Valsartan	Diovan	40 – 160mg	14.76 – 21.66

Beta blockers

Generic name	Proprietary name(s)	Daily dose range	NHS cost for 28 days (£)	Comments
Acebutolol	Sectral	400 – 800mg in 2 doses	19.19 – 37.24	Cardioselective (relatively) ISA
Atenolol	Tenormin	50mg	1.02 (generic) 5.11 (proprietary)	Cardioselective Water-soluble
Bisoprolol fumarate	Cardicor, Emcor, Monocor	5 – 20mg	1.68 – 5.38 (generic) 7.96 – 18.84 (proprietary)	Cardioselective
Carvedilol	Eucardic	12.5 – 50mg	9.07 – 22.18 (generic) 9.35 – 23.36 (proprietary)	Arteriolar vasodilator
Celiprolol hydrochloride	Celectol	200 – 400mg	8.11 – 19.21 (generic) 16.28 – 32.56 (proprietary)	Water-soluble, ISA, Arteriolar vasodilator
Labetalol hydrochloride	Trandate	100 – 800mg in 2 doses	3.79 – 19.10 (generic) 3.79 – 9.42 (proprietary)	Arteriolar vasodilator
Metoprolol tartrate	Betaloc, Lopresor	100-200mg in 1-2 doses	2.41 – 3.84 (generic) 1.72 – 6.68 (proprietary)	Cardioselective
Nadolol	Corgard	80 – 240mg	5.20 – 15.60	Water-soluble
Nebivolol	Nebilet	2.5 – 5mg	4.62 – 9.23	Cardioselective, Arteriolar vasodilator
Oxprenolol hydrochloride	Trasicor	80 – 320mg in 2 -3 doses	3.11 – 6.61 (generic) 3.11 –12.40 (proprietary)	ISA
Pindolol	Visken	10 – 45 mg in 2 – 3 doses	4.88 – 21.99	ISA
Propranolol	Beta-Prograne, Inderal LA,	160 – 320mg in 2 doses	1.45 – 3.88 (generic) 5.40 – 13.34 (proprietary)	
Timolol	Betim	5 – 60mg	0.97 – 11.65	

Calcium channel blockers (CCB) (see also the relevant discussion in Chapter 5)

Generic name	Proprietary name(s)	Daily dose range	NHS cost for 28 days (£)	Comments
Amlodipine besilate	Istin	5 – 10mg	2.51 – 2.93 (generic) 13.04 – 19.47 (proprietary)	
Diltiazem hydrochloride	Adizem-XL, Angitil-SR or XL, Calcicard-CR, Dilcardia-SR, Dilzem, Slozem, Tildiem, Viazem, Zemtard	180 – 360mg	Many prices (see latest MIMS)	BNF recommends brand prescribing for longer-acting formulations
Felodipine	Plendil	2.5 – 20mg	6.70 – 24.02	
Isradipine	Prescal	2.5 – 10mg in 2 doses	7.52 – 30.08	
Lacidipine	Motens	2 – 6mg	10.23 – 25.53	
Lercanidipine hydrochloride	Zanadip	10 – 20mg	5.80 – 11.60	
Nicardipine hydrochloride	Cardene, Cardene SR	60 – 120mg in 3 doses (2 doses if sustained release)	13.38 – 26.76 (generic) 10.21 – 25.71 (proprietary)	
Nifedipine	Adalat, Adipine MR, Cardilate MR, Coracten, Fortipine LA, Tensipine MR	20 – 80mg in 1 – 2 doses	3.99 – 16.00	Only sustained release preparations are suitable for hypertension
Nisoldipine	Syscor MR	10 – 40mg daily	8.77 – 35.08	
Verapamil hydrochloride	Cordilox, Securon	240 – 480mg in 2 – 3 doses	2.52– 9.35 (generic) 5.87 – 12.58 (proprietary)	

Thiazide and thiazide-like diuretics

Generic name	Proprietary name(s)	Daily dose range	NHS cost for 28 days (£)
Bendroflumethiazide	various	2.5mg in the morning	1.04 (generic) 1.53 - 2.00 (proprietary)
Chlortalidone	Hygroton	25 – 50mg in the morning	0.82 – 1.64
Cyclopenthiazide	Navidrex	250 – 500 microgrammes in the morning	0.64 – 1.27
Indapamide	Natrilix	2.5mg in the morning	3.69 (generic) 4.20 (proprietary)
Indapamide SR	Natrilix SR	1.5mg in the morning	4.20
Metolazone	Metenix 5	5mg in the morning	5.70
Xipamide	Diurexan	20mg in the morning	3.89

Alpha 1 adrenergic blockers

Generic name	Proprietary name(s)	Daily dose range	NHS cost for 28 days (£)
Doxazosin	Cardura	1 – 16mg	1.81 – 18.32 (generic) 10.56 – 112.64 (proprietary)
	Cardura XL (modified release)	4 – 8mg	6.34 – 12.67 (modified release)
Indoramin	Baratol	50 – 200mg in 2-3 doses	6.00 – 24.00
Prazosin	Hypovase	1.5mg in 3 doses to 20mg	2.87– 17.50 (generic) 3.76 – 21.95 (proprietary)
Terazosin	Hytrin	1 – 20mg at bedtime	3.54 – 51.94 (generic) 2.29 – 34.28 (proprietary)

Aldosterone antagonist

Generic name	Proprietary name(s)	Daily dose range	NHS cost for 28 days (£)
Spionolactone	Aldactone	12.5mg	1.50 (generic) 1.24 (proprietary)

Other antihypertensive agents

Generic name	Proprietary name(s)	Daily dose range	NHS cost for 28 days (£)
Hydralazine	Apresoline	50 – 100mg in 2 doses	3.31 – 6.62 (generic) 1.67 – 3.33
Minoxidil	Loniten	2.5 – 50mg	4.14 – 71.59
Clonidine	Catapres	1.5 – 3mg in 3 doses	2.35 – 4.70
Methyldopa	Aldomet	500mg in 2 doses to 3000mg in 3 doses	3.01 – 14.04 (generic) 1.75 – 10.64 (proprietary)
Moxonidine	Physiotens	200mcg in 1 dose to 600mcg in 2 doses	9.72 – 22.98

Combination antihypertensive agents

Proprietary name	Constituents	Description	Daily dose range	NHS cost for 28 days (£)
Accuretic	Quinapril 10mg/ Hydrochlorothiazide 12.5mg	ACE/thiazide diuretic	1 – 2	11.75 – 23.50
Acezide	Captopril 50mg/ Hydrochlorothiazide 25mg	ACE/thiazide diuretic	1 – 2	13.15 – 26.30
Amil-Co	Amiloride 5mg/ Hydrochlorothiazide 50mg	Potassium sparing diuretic/ thiazide diuretic	1 – 4	1.95 – 7.80
Beta-Adalat	Atenolol 50mg/ Nifedipine 20mg	Beta blocker/CCB	1 – 2	10.41 – 20.82
Capozide	Captopril 50mg/ Hydrochlorothiazide 25mg	ACE/thiazide diuretic	1	13.15
Capozide LS	Captopril 25mg/ Hydrochlorothiazide 12.5mg	ACE/thiazide diuretic	1	10.46
Carace 10 Plus	Lisinopril 10mg/ Hydrochlorothiazide 12.5mg	ACE/thiazide diuretic	1 – 2	10.51 – 21.02
Carace 20 Plus	Lisinopril 20mg/ Hydrochlorothiazide 12.5mg	ACE/thiazide diuretic	1 – 2	11.89 – 23.78
Co-Betaloc	Metoprolol 100mg/ Hydrochlorothiazide 12.5mg	Beta blocker/ thiazide diuretic	1 – 3 in 1 – 3 doses	5.59 – 16.77
Co-Diovan	Valsartan 80 or 160mg/ Hydrochlorothiazide 12.5 or 25mg as 80/12.5, 160/12.5 or 160/25	ARB/thiazide diuretic	1	16.44 – 21.66
Coversyl Plus	Perindopril 4mg/ Indapamide 1.25mg	ACE/diuretic	1 in the morning	13.96
Dyazide	Triamterene 50mg/ Hydrochlorothiazide 25mg	Potassium sparing diuretic/ thiazide diuretic	1	0.89
Innozide	Enalapril 20mg/ Hydrochlorothiazide 12.5mg	ACE/thiazide diuretic	1 – 2	13.90 – 27.80

Proprietary name	Constituents	Description	Daily dose range	NHS cost for 28 days (£)
Kalspare	Chlortalidone 50mg/ Triamterene 50mg	Thiazide diuretic/ potassium sparing diuretic	1 - 2	3.05 – 6.10
Kalten	Atenolol 50mg/ Hydrochlorothiazide 25mg/ Amiloride 2.5mg	ACE/thiazide diuretic/potassium sparing diuretic	1	8.39
Micardis Plus	Telmisartan 40 or 80mg/ Hydrochlorothiazide 12.5mg	ARB/thiazide diuretic	1	11.34 – 14.18
Moduret 25	Amiloride 2.5mg/ Hydrochlorothiazide 25mg	Potassium sparing diuretic/thiazide diuretic	1 – 4 in divided doses	1.72 – 6.88
Moduretic	Amiloride 5mg/ Hydrochlorothiazide 50mg	Potassium sparing diuretic/ thiazide diuretic	1/2 to 2	1.04 – 4.16
Navispare	Cyclopenthiazide 0.25mg/ Amiloride 2.5mg	Thiazide diuretic/ potassium sparing diuretic	1 - 2	2.25 – 4.50
Secadrex	Acebutolol 200mg/ Hydrochlorothiazide 12.5mg	Beta blocker/ thiazide diuretic	1 – 2	17.59 – 35.18
Tenif	Atenolol 50mg/ Nifedipine 20mg	Beta blocker/ CCB	1 – 2	10.63 – 21.26
Tenoret 50	Atenolol 50mg/ Chlortalidone 12.5mg	Beta blocker/ thiazide diuretic	1	5.70
Tenoretic	Atenolol 100mg/ Chlortalidone 25mg	Beta blocker/ thiazide diuretic	1	8.12
Trasidrex	Oxprenolol 160mg/ Cyclopenthiazide 0.25mg	Beta blocker/ thiazide diuretic	1-2	8.88 – 17.76
Triam-Co	Triamterene 50mg/ Hydrochlorothiazide 25mg	Potassium sparing diuretic/ thiazide diuretic	1	1.58
Zestoretic 10	Lisinopril 10mg/ Hydrochlorothiazide 12.5mg	ACE/ thiazide diuretic	1- 2	13.01 – 26.02
Zestoretic 20	Lisinopril 20mg/ Hydrochlorothiazide 12.5mg	ACE/ thiazide diuretic	1 - 2	14.72

Lipid-regulating drugs

Anion-exchange resins

Generic name	Proprietary name(s)	Daily dose range	NHS cost for 28 days (£)
Colestyramine	Questran	1 – 9 sachets	9.83 – 88.45
Colestipol hydrochloride	Colestid	5 – 30g daily in 1 or 2 doses	14.05 – 84.28

Fibrates

Generic name	Proprietary name(s)	Daily dose range	NHS cost for 28 days (£)
Bezafibrate	Bezalip,	600mg in 3 doses	7.85 (generic) 7.69 (proprietary)
	Bezalip Mono	400mg in 1 dose	7.55 (Mono)
Ciprofibrate	Modalim	100mg	14.72
Fenofibrate	Lipantil micro, Supralip mono	134 – 267mg	14.23 (generic) 14.50 – 21.75 (proprietary)
Gemfibrozil	Lopoid	1.2 – 1.5g daily in 2 divided doses	28.27 – 35.34 (generic) 35.57 – 44.46 (proprietary)

Statins

Generic name	Proprietary name(s)	Daily dose range	NHS cost for 28 days (£)
Atorvastatin	Lipitor	10 – 80mg at night	18.03 – 28.21
Fluvastatin	Lescol	20 – 80mg at night	12.72 – 16.00
Pravastatin sodium	Lipostat	10 – 40mg at night	3.42 – 6.55 (generic) 15.05 – 27.61 (proprietary)
Rosuvastatin	Crestor	10 – 40mg	18.03 – 29.69
Simvastatin	Zocor	10 – 80mg at night	2.12 – 26.79 (generic) 18.03 – 29.69 (proprietary)

Azetidinones

Generic name	Proprietary name(s)	Daily dose range	NHS cost for 28 days (£)
Ezetimibe	Ezetrol	10mg	26.31

Nicotinic acid group

Generic name	Proprietary name(s)	Daily dose range	NHS cost for 28 days (£)
Acipimox	Olbetam	500 – 750mg in divided doses	28.83 – 43.24
Nicotinic acid	Niaspan (modified release)	1 – 2g (modified release)	17.25 – 29.50

Fish oils

Generic name	Proprietary name(s)	Daily dose range	NHS cost for 28 days (£)
Omega-3-acid ethyl esters	Omacor	1 – 4 capsules	13.89 – 55.56
Omega-3-marine triglycerides	Maxepa	5 capsules twice daily OR 5ml twice daily	38.19 19.10

Blood glucose-lowering drugs

Sulphonylureas

Generic name	Proprietary name(s)	Daily dose range	NHS cost for 28 days (£)	Comments
Tolbutamide		250 – 2000mg	1.20 – 9.56	Short-acting
Gliclazide	Diamicron	40 – 320mg (160mg maximum single dose)	0.76 – 6.08 (generic) 1.52 – 12.15 (proprietary)	Excreted in bile
Gliclazide MR	Diamicron MR	30 – 120mg, in the morning	4.40 – 17.60	Increments at 2 week intervals
Glipizide	Glibenese, Minodiab	2.5 – 20mg (15mg maximum single dose)	1.48– 8.72	Before breakfast or lunch
Glimepiride	Amaryl at breakfast	1 – 6mg,	4.51 – 22.24	
Gliquidone	Glurenorm	15 – 180mg (60 mg maximum single dose)	2.46 – 29.47	
Glibenclamide	Daonil, Euglycon	2.5 – 15mg	1.06 – 2.88 (generic) 1.73 – 8.07 (proprietary)	Long-acting
Chlorpropamide		100 – 500mg	2.38 – 5.60	Interacts with alcohol, Avoid in elderly

Post-prandial regulators of glucose

Generic name	Proprietary name(s)	Daily dose range	NHS cost for 28 days (£)	Comments
Repaglinide	NovoNorm	0.5 – 16mg (4mg maximum single dose) before meals	3.66 – 29.27	Not recommended in over 75 years of age
Nateglinide	Starlix	180 – 540mg in 3 divided doses	19.75 – 22.50	Licenced only in combination with metformin

Biguanide

Generic name	Proprietary name(s)	Daily dose range	NHS cost for 28 days (£)
Metformin	Glucophage	500 – 2000mg in divided doses	1.41 – 2.79 (generic) 0.80 – 3.20 (proprietary)

Thiazolidinediones

Generic name	Proprietary name(s)	Daily dose range	NHS cost for 28 days (£)	Comments
Pioglitazone	Actos	15 – 45mg	24.14 – 36.96	Monitor LFTs
Rosiglitazone	Avandia	4 – 8mg	24.74 – 50.78	Monitor LFTs; can increase dose after 8 weeks

Other blood glucose-lowering drugs

Generic name	Proprietary name(s)	Daily dose range	NHS cost for 28 days (£)
Acarbose	Glucobay	50 – 600mg	2.05 – 21.02

Combination antihypertensive agents

Proprietary name	Constituents	Description	Daily dose range	NHS cost for 28 days (£)
Avandamet	2/1000: rosiglitazone 2mg + metformin 1000mg	Thiazolidinedione/ Biguanide	1 tablet twice daily	27.71
	4/1000: rosiglitazone 4mg + metformin 1000mg		1 tablet twice daily	52.45
	2/500: rosglitazone 2mg + metformin 500mg		2 tablets twice daily	52.45

Appendix 2
National Service Framework Standards for Diabetes

Department of Health:National Service Framework for Diabetes Standards.
(London, HMSO, 2001)

Standard
1. *Prevention:* To reduce the number of people who develop type 2 diabetes
2. *Diagnosis:* To ensure that people with diabetes are identified as early as possible
3. *Empowerment:* To ensure that people with diabetes are empowered to enhance their personal control over the day-to-day management of their diabetes in a way that enables them to experience the best quality of life
4. *Clinical Care:* To maximise the quality of life of all people with diabetes and to reduce their risk of developing the long-term complications of diabetes
5. *Young People With Diabetes:* high quality care
6. *Young People With Diabetes:* smooth transition from paediatric to adult services
7. *Diabetic Emergencies:* To minimise the impact on people with diabetes of the acute complications of diabetes
8. *Hospital Admissions:* Not relevant to primary care
9. *Diabetes And Pregnancy:* Rarely relevant to primary care
10. *Detection And Management Of Long-Term Complications:* All patients with diabetes receive regular surveillance for the long-term complications of diabetes
11. *Detection And Management Of Long-Term Complications:* Implement and monitor agreed protocols of care so that all those who develop complications receive appropriate care
12. *Detection And Management Of Long-Term Complications:* All those requiring multi-agency support will receive integrated health and social care

Appendix 3
New GMS Contract Indicators for Diabetes

General Practice Committee: The New GP Contract Indicators for Diabetes (2004 – 2006)

Indicator	Points	Maximum threshold
DM1: The practice can produce a register of all patients with diabetes mellitus	6	Not applicable
DM2: The percentage of patients with diabetes whose notes record BMI in the previous 12 months	3	90%
DM3: The percentage of patients with diabetes in whom there is a record of smoking status in the previous 15 months except those who have never smoked where smoking status should be recorded once	3	90%
DM4: The percentage of patients with diabetes who smoke and whose notes contain a record that smoking cessation advice has been offered in the last 15 months	5	90%
DM5: The percentage of diabetic patients who have a record of HbA1c or equivalent in the previous 15 months	3	90%
DM6: The percentage of patients with diabetes in whom the last HbA1c is 7.4 or less (or equivalent test / reference range depending on local laboratory) in last 15 months	16	50%
DM7: The percentage of patients with diabetes in whom the last HbA1c is 10 or less (or equivalent test / reference range depending on local laboratory) in last 15 months	11	85%
DM8: The percentage of diabetic patients who have a record of retinal screening in the previous 15 months	5	90%
DM9: The percentage of patients with diabetes with a record of presence or absence of peripheral pulses in the previous 15 months	3	90%
DM10: The percentage of patients with diabetes with a record of neuropathy testing in the previous 15 months	3	90%
DM11: The percentage of patients with diabetes who have a record of the blood pressure in the past 15 months	3	90%
DM12: The percentage of patients with diabetes in whom the last blood pressure is 145/85 or less	17	55%
DM13: The percentage of patients with diabetes who have a record of micro-albuminuria testing in the previous 15 months (exception reporting for patients with proteinuria)	3	90%

Indicator	Points	Maximum threshold
DM14: The percentage of patients with diabetes who have a record of serum creatinine testing in the previous 15 months	3	90%
DM15: The percentage of patients with diabetes with proteinuria or micro-albuminuria who are treated with ACE inhibitors (or A2 antagonists)	3	70%
DM16: The percentage of patients with diabetes who have a record of total cholesterol in the previous 15 months	3	90%
DM17: The percentage of patients with diabetes whose last measured total cholesterol within previous 15 months is 5 mmol/l or less	6	60%
DM18: The percentage of patients with diabetes who have had influenza immunisation in the preceding 1 September to 31 March	3	85%

NB: All minimum thresholds are 25%

These indicators are due for review in 2005 – 2006, and may change for the following two financial year cycle.

Appendix 4
Further reading and useful contacts

In a rapidly changing field, keeping up-to-date is likely to involve regular perusal of suitable internet sites and journals. The author recommends the following as starting points for those wishing to keep abreast of developments in this field:

Books

The following books discuss much of what is covered in this book, but in greater depth:

- Bailey CJ, Krentz AJ. *Type 2 Diabetes in Practice*. 2nd Edition. London: Royal Society of Medicine Press Limited, 2005.

- Levene LS. *Management of Type 2 Diabetes Mellitus in Primary Care: A Practical Guide*. Edinburgh: Butterworth Heinemann, 2003.

- MacKinnon M. *Providing Diabetes Care in General Practice: A Practical Guide for the Primary Care Team*. 4th Edition. London: Class Publishing, 2002.

- Williams B. *Diabetes and Hypertension: A Fatal Attraction Explained*. Beckenham: Publishing Initiatives Books, 1996.

Journals

- *Practical Diabetes International* is published every two months and is excellent. PMH Publications, PO BOX 100, Chichester, West Sussex, PO18 8HD, mail it free on request to health care professionals.

- *Diabetes Digest* is also very useful for keeping up to date with diabetes literature. It is published quarterly in the UK for health care professionals with an interest in diabetes and can be obtained from SB Communications Group, 15 Mandeville Courtyard, 142 Battersea Park Road, London SW11 4NB; telephone 020-7627 1510; e-mail: info@sbcommunicationsgroup.com.

- Important research and reviews about diabetes may be published in eminent peer-reviewed journals with wide circulation, such as the *British Medical Journal*, the *Lancet*, or *The New England Journal of Medicine*, or those with specialist interest, such as *Diabetes Care*, *Diabetic Medicine*, or *Diabetologica*. These are either available on subscription or are held in any self-respecting hospital postgraduate library.

Electronic Resources

Traditional textbooks fail frequently to incorporate newly published research. Furthermore, textbooks may lack specific references, selected according to explicit principles of evidence, to support their declarations about diagnosis and management. Electronic evidence databases, available either via the Internet or on CD-ROM, are regarded as being better able to overcome these drawbacks. No single database will address all needs. A comprehensive search needs to choose an effective strategy that will look at several appropriate databases. Try contacting the local postgraduate medical library to cultivate the medical librarian and to book a training session: it is well worth it! Another invaluable benefit from contacting the local postgraduate library is obtaining a personal ATHENS (Access To Higher Education via NISS authentication System) username and password. This allows the user to access for free many otherwise remote or pay-to-view electronic resources. Every effort has been made to ensure that the web addresses cited below are accurate at the time of printing. If these change, browsers may be redirected to the new webpage, or there is always Google.

A good starting point for any electronic searches is the National Electronic Library of Health (NeLH), which is well organised and has excellent links It is available free both to NHS staff via the NHSNet and to the general public; online: www.nelh.nhs.uk/. The NeLH has just launched its diabetes specialist library, online: http://libraries.nelh.nhs.uk/diabetes/

The following databases are useful:

- Many, but not all, medical articles are indexed in the massive **Medline** database, compiled by the National Library of Medicine in the United States. There is no filtering on the original Medline, so each article needs to be evaluated critically. Free access to Medline has been available since 1997 via PubMed, online: http://www.ncbi.nih.gov/entrez/query.fcgi.

- **AMED** (Allied and Complimentary Medicine Database) is a unique bibliographic database produced by the Health Care Information Service of the British Library. It covers a selection of journals in three separate subject areas, several professions allied to medicine, complementary medicine and palliative care. NHS professionals in England and Wales have free access to AMED via the NHSNet. Further details are available, online: http://www.bl.uk/collections/health/amed.html

- The **Cochrane Library** is a collection of databases, updated quarterly, which include systematic reviews and registers of controlled trials. Many researchers now favour Cochrane when starting a literature search. It can be obtained on a subscription basis, either on CD-ROM or via the Internet, from Update Software Ltd., Summertown, Pavilion, Middle Way, Oxford, OX2 7LG. Tel (01865) 513902 or Web: http://www.cochrane.org/index2.htm or E-mail: info@update.co.uk The Cochrane Database of Systematic Reviews is an important information source for the effectiveness of treatments. It is available free to NHS staff via the knowledge section of the NeLH, online: www.nelh.nhs.uk/ and the abstracts are free to all via: http://www.update-software.com/publications/cochrane/

- Several free related databases are available online: http://www.york.ac.uk/inst/crd/crddatabases.htm
  - **DARE** (the database of abstracts of reviews of effectiveness)
  - **NHS EED** (the NHS economic evaluation database)
  - **HTA** (health technology assessment)

- **TRIP** is a free database that searches over 55 sites of high quality medical information, online: http://www.tripdatabase.com/ Free access can be obtained by logging in via ATHENS.

Organisations

Many organisations have their own web sites with useful information:

- The American Diabetes Association (ADA) publishes comprehensive and referenced clinical practice recommendations that are up-dated annually, available: http://www.diabetes.org.

- Diabetes UK caters not only for health care professionals, but also for patients and other interested lay people, at 10 Parkway, London NW1 7AA, telephone (020) 7424 1000 (GPs and practice nurses can join the Primary Care section). It does post guidance on its website. Online. Available: http://www.diabetes.org.uk

- The Department of Health (DoH), for finding official documents: http://www.dh.gov.uk/Home/fs/en

- National Institute for Health and Clinical Excellence (NICE) has guidelines on various aspects of diabetes in support of the Diabetes NSF and on hypertension in 2004, and guidance, particularly on new treatments. Online. Available: http://www.nice.org.uk

- The Scottish Intercollegiate Guidelines Network (SIGN) published in November 2001 its own guidelines for the management of diabetes (guideline number 55). Their evidence base is very well set out and it carries an extensive list of references. They can be downloaded from the SIGN website: http://www.sign.ac.uk/

- The Science and Education Department of the British Medical Association (BMA) produced in February 2004 a useful guide for healthcare professionals managing patients with diabetes. It is downloadable as a PDF from the BMA website, online: http://www.bma.org.uk/ap.nsf/Content/Diabetes?OpenDocument&Highlight=2,diabetes

- The University of Warwick's "Warwick Diabetes Care" was launched in November 2000. It is an extremely useful point of contact for all providers of diabetic care through educational courses, support of diabetes research, and practical resources and links. It can be contacted via telephone (024)7657 2958 or e-mail: diabetes@warwick.ac.uk. Its website is http://www2.warwick.ac.uk/fac/med/healthcom/diabetes/

- The Department of Health's Medicines and Healthcare products Regulatory Agency (MHRA) is a very useful source of information about medical equipment. Similarly to the yellow card reporting system for adverse drug reactions, the MHRA requests practitioners to report adverse incidents involving medical devices. Obtaining further information or reporting an adverse incident can be done via the MHRA website: www.mhra.gov.uk

Appendix 5
Abbreviations and acronyms

4S, Scandinavian Simvastatin Survival Study

ABCD, Appropriate Blood Pressure Control in Diabetes/Association of British Clinical Diabetologists

ACE, angiotensin converting enzyme

ACR, albumin-creatinine ratio

ADA, American Diabetes Association

ADDITION, Anglo-Danish-Dutch Study of Intensive Treatment in People with Screen Detected Diabetes in Primary Care

ADOPT, A Diabetes Outcome Progression Trial

AER, albumin excretion rate

AF, atrial fibrillation

AGEs, advanced glycosylation end products

AIC, Adverse Incident Centre

ALLHAT, Antihypertensive and Lipid Lowering to prevent Heart Attack Trial

AMED, Allied and Complimentary Medicine Database

ARB, angiotensin II receptor antagonists

ARR, absolute risk reduction

ASCOT, Anglo-Scandinavian Cardiac Outcomes Trial

BHF, British Heart Foundation

BHS, British Hypertension Society

BMI, body mass index

BNF, British National Formulary

CAN, cardiac autonomic neuropathy

CAPP, Captopril Prevention Project

CARDS, Collaborative Atorvastatin Diabetes Study

CARE, cholesterol and recurrent events trial

CBT, cognitive behaviour therapy

CHD, coronary heart disease

CNS, central nervous system

CVA, cerebrovascular accident

CVD, cardiovascular disease

CPK, creatine phosphokinase

DAFNE, dose adjustment for normal eating randomised controlled trial

DARE, the database of abstracts of reviews of effectiveness

DASH, Dietary Approaches to Stop Hypertension

DCCT, Diabetes Control and Complications Trial

DECODE, Diabetes Epidemiology: Collaborative Analysis of Diagnostic Criteria in Europe

DESMOND, Diabetes Education for Self-Management: Ongoing and Newly Diagnosed

ECG, electrocardiogram

EMEA, European Medicines Agency

EUROPA, EURopean trial On reduction of cardiac events with Perindopril in stable coronary Artery disease

FACET, Fosinopril versus Amlodipine Cardiovascular Events Randomised Trial

FIELD, Fenofibrate Intervention and Event Lowering in Diabetes study

G, grammes

GI, glycaemic index

GMS, General Medical Services

HbA1c, Haemoglobin A1c (glycosylated haemoglobin)

HDFP, Hypertension Detection and Follow-up Program

HDL, high density lipoprotein

HOPE, Heart Outcomes Prevention Evaluation Study

HOT, Hypertension Optimal Treatment Trial

HTA, health technology assessment
IDF, International Diabetes Federation
INVEST, International Verapamil-Trandolapril Study
INR, international normalised ratio
ISA, intrinsic sympathomimetic activity
LDL, low density lipoprotein
LIFE, Losartan Intervention for Endpoint reduction in hypertension study
LIPID, Long-Term Intervention with Pravastatin in Ischaemic Disease Study
LV, left ventricle or left ventricular
LVH, left ventricular hypertrophy
MCV, mean corpuscular volume
MHRA, Medicines and Healthcare products Regulatory Agency
MI, myocardial infarction
MIMS, Monthly Index of Medical Specialities
MNT, medical nutritional therapy
MRC, Medical Research Council
MRFIT, Multiple Risk Factor Intervention Trial
NCEP, National Cholesterol Education Program
NHS EED, the NHS economic evaluation database
NICE, National Institute of Clinical Excellence
NNT, number needed to treat
NORDIL, Nordic Diltiazem Study
NRT, nicotine replacement therapy

NSF, National Service Framework
QALY, Quality Adjusted Life Years
QOF, Quality Outcomes Framework
PMS, Personal Medical Services
PROactive, Prospective Pioglitazone Clinical Trial in Macrovascular Events
PROCAM, Prospective Cardiovascular Munster Study
PVD, peripheral vascular disease
RCT, randomised controlled trial
RECORD, Rosiglitazone Evaluated for Cardiac Outcomes and Regulation of Glycaemia in Diabetes study
SHEP, Systolic Hypertension in the Elderly Program
SIGN, Scottish Intercollegiate Guidelines Network
STOP-2, Swedish Trial in Old Patients with Hypertension
SYST-EUR, Systolic Hypertension in Europe Trial
SYST-CHINA, Systolic Hypertension in China
TC, total cholesterol
TG, triglyceride
UKPDS, United Kingdom Prospective Diabetes Study
VLCD, very low calorie diet
VLDL, very low density lipoprotein
WHO, World Health Organisation
WHR, waist hip ratio

References

Chapter 1 references

1: Semenkovich CF, Heinecke JW. The mystery of diabetes and atherosclerosis: time for a new plot. *Diabetes* 1997; **46**: 327-334.

2: Howlett HCS, Bailey CJ in Krentz AJ (Ed.). *Drug Treatment of Type 2 Diabetes.* Auckland: ADIS International, 2000.

3: Currie CJ, *et al*. NHS acute sector expenditure for diabetes: the present, future, and excess in-patient cost of care. *Diab Med* 1997; **14:** 686-692.

4: British Diabetic Association, King's Fund, Economists Advisory Group and SmithKline Beecham Pharmaceuticals UK, 2000. T2ARDIS: Implications for Seamless Care Provision in Type 2 Diabetes in the UK. Data presented at the Diabetes UK Professional Conference, 2000.

5: Department of Health. National Service Framework for Diabetes: Standards. London: HMSO, 2001.

6: Department of Health. National Service Framework for Diabetes: Delivery strategy. London: HMSO, 2002.

7: General Practice Committee. The New GP Contract. GPC 2003.

Chapter 2 references

1: Simmons D. Prevention of Complications: A Commentary. In Williams R, Herman W, Kinmouth A-L, *et al*, editors. *The Evidence Base for Diabetes Care.* Chichester: John Wiley & Sons, Ltd, 2002.

2: Stamler J, Vaccaro O, Neaton JD, Wentworth D. Diabetes, other risk factors, and 12-yr cardiovascular mortality for men screened in the Multiple Risk Factor Intervention Trial. *Diab Care* 1993; **16**: 433-444.

3: Barrett-Connor EL, *et al*. Why is diabetes mellitus a stronger risk factor for fatal ischemic heart disease in women than in men? The Rancho Bernardo Study. *J Am Med Assoc* 1991; **265**: 627-633.

4: Abstract presented by Woodward M *et al* at the Second International Conference on Women, Heart Disease and Stroke, Orlando, FL February 2005.In *Circulation* 2005 **111**: e40-e88.

5: Wingard DL, Barrett-Connor E, Wedick E. What is the Evidence that Changing Tobacco Use Reduces the Incidence of Diabetic Complications? In Williams R, Herman W, Kinmouth A-L, *et al*, editors. *The Evidence Base for Diabetes Care*. Chichester: John Wiley & Sons, Ltd, 2002.

6: Hatziandreu EI, Koplan JP, Weinstein MC, *et al*. A cost-effectiveness analysis of exercise as a health-promotion activity. *Am J Public Health* 1988; **78**: 1417-1421.

7: Department of Health. At Least Five a Week: evidence on the impact of physical activity and its relationship to health. A report from the Chief Medical Officer. London: HMSO, 2004.

8: Department of Health. Health Survey for England 2003: Trends. Department of Health 2004. Online, available: http://www.dh.gov.uk

9: Lewington S, Clarke R, Qizilbash N, Peto R, Collins R; Prospective Studies Collaboration. Age-specific relevance of usual blood pressure to vascular mortality: a meta-analysis of individual data for one million adults in 61 prospective studies. *Lancet* 2002; **360**: 1902-1913.

10: Ezzati M, Lopez AD, Rogers A, Vander Hoorn S, Murray CJ; Comparative Risk Assessment Collaborating Group. Selected major risk factors and global and regional burden of disease. *Lancet* 2002; **360**: 1347-1360.

11: Scottish Intercollegiate Guidelines Network (SIGN) 1997. Management of Diabetic Cardiovascular Disease, 1-22. Available. Online: http://www.sign.ac.uk

12: Dawson KG, McKenzie JK, Ross SA, *et al*. Hypertension and Diabetes. *Can Med Assoc J* 1993; **149**: 821-826.

13: Gerstein HC. Glucose: a continuous risk factor for cardiovascular disease. *Diab Med* 1997; **14**: S25-S31.

14: The Diabetes Control and Complications Trial Research Group. The effect of intensive treatment of diabetes on the development and progression of long-term complications in insulin-dependent diabetes mellitus. *N Engl J Med* 1993; **329**: 977-986.

15: Stratton IM, Adler AI, Neil HA, *et al*. Association of glycaemia with macrovascular and microvascular complications of type 2 diabetes (UKPDS 35). United Kingdom Prospective Diabetes Study Group. *Br Med J* 2000; **321**: 405-412.

16: Valmadrid CT, Klein R, Moses SE, *et al*. Alcohol intake and the risk of coronary heart disease mortality in persons with older onset diabetes mellitus. *J Am Med Assoc* 1999; **282**: 239-246.

17: Ajani UA, Gaziano JM, Lotufo PA, *et al*. Alcohol consumption and risk of coronary heart disease by diabetes status. *Circulation* 2000; **102**: 500-505.

18: Sacco RL, Elkind M, Boden-Albala B, *et al*. The protective effect of moderate alcohol consumption on ischaemic stroke. *J Am Med* Assoc 1999; **282**: 53-60.

19: Mayne EE. Haemostatic disorders in diabetes mellitus. In: Stout RW ed. *Diabetes and Atherosclerosis*. Dordrecht: Kluwer Academic Publishers, 1992: 219-235.

20: Meade TW, Mellows S, Brozovic M, Miller GJ, Chakrabarti RR, North WR, *et al*. Haemostatic function and ischaemic heart disease: principal results of the Northwick Park Heart Study. *Lancet* 1986; **ii**: 533-537.

21: Yarnell JW, Baker IA, Sweetnam PM, Bainton D, O'Brien JR, Whitehead PJ, *et al*. Fibrinogen, viscosity and white cell count are major risk factors for ischaemic heart disease. The Caerphilly and Speedwell Collaborative Heart Disease Studies. *Circulation* 1991; **83**: 836-844.

22: Hayes JR. Non-ischaemic heart disease in diabetes mellitus. In: Stout RW ed. *Diabetes and Atherosclerosis*. Dordrecht: Kluwer Academic Publishers, 1992: 255-265.

23: Naas AA, Davidson NC, Thompson C, Cummings F, Ogston SA, Jung RT, *et al*. QT and QTc dispersion are accurate predictors of cardiac death in newly diagnosed non-insulin dependent diabetes: cohort study. *Br Med J* 1998; **316**: 745-746.

24: O'Brien IA, McFadden JP, Corrall RJM. The influence of autonomic neuropathy on mortality in insulin-dependent diabetes. *Q J Med* 1991; **79**: 495-502.

25: Pai JK, Pischon T, Ma J, *et al*. Inflammatory Markers and the Risk of Coronary Heart Disease in Men and Women. *N Engl J Med* 2004; **351**: 2599-2610.

26: Gilbert RE, Cooper ME, McNally PG, O'Brien RC, Taft J, Jerums G. Microalbuminuria: prognostic and therapeutic implications in diabetes mellitus. *Diab Med* 1994; **11**: 636-645.

27: Gerstein HC, Mann JF, Yi Q, Zinman B, Dineen SF, Hoogwerf B, Halle JP, Young J, Rashkow A, Joyce C, Nawaaz S, Yusuf S. Albuminuria and risk of cardiovascular events, death, and heart failure in diabetic and nondiabetic individuals. *J Am Med Assoc* 2001 July 25; **286 (4)**: 421-426.

28: Lunetta M, Infantone L, Calogero AE, Infantone E. Increased urinary albumin excretion is a marker of risk for retinopathy and coronary heart disease in patients with type 2 diabetes. *Diab Res Clin Pract* 1998 April; **40 (1)**: 45-51.

29: Dinneen SF, Gerstein HC. The association of microalbuminuria and mortality in non-insulin-dependent diabetes mellitus. *Arch Intern Med* 1997; **157(13)**: 1413-8.

30: MacLeod JM, Lutale J, Marshall SM. Albumin excretion and vascular deaths in NIDDM. *Diabetologia* 1995; **38(5)**: 610-6.

31: Carr DB, Ulzschneider KM, Hull RL, *et al*. Intra-abdominal fat is a major determinant of the National Cholesterol Education Program Adult Treatment Panel III criteria for the metabolic syndrome. *Diabetes* 2004; **53(8)**:2087-2094.

32: International Diabetes Federation press release, 14 April 2005. Online. Available: http://www.idf.org/home/index.cfm?unode=32EF2063-B966-468F-928C-A5682A4E3910

33: Hanif MW *et al*. Obesity is highly prevalent in Indo-Asians with metabolic syndrome. *Diabetes* 2002; **19 (Supplement 2)**: 33.

Chapter 3 references

1: Winocour PH, Fisher M. Prediction of cardiovascular risk in people with diabetes. *Diab Med* 2003; **20**: 515-527.

2: American Diabetes Association: Position Statement. Standards of Medical Care in Diabetes. *Diab Care* 2005; **28 (Supplement 1)**: S4-S36.

3: North of England Hypertension Guideline Development Group. Evidence-based Clinical Practice Guideline: Essential hypertension: managing adults in primary care. London: HMSO National Institute of Clinical Excellence, August 2004. Available. Online via NICE

4: Assmann G, Schulte H. The Prospective Cardiovascular Munster (PROCAM) Study: prevalence of hyperlipidemia in persons with hypertension and/or diabetes and their relationship to coronary heart disease. *Am Heart J* 1988; **116**: 1713-1724.

5: Menotti A, Puddu PE, Lanti M. Comparison of the Framingham risk-function based coronary chart with risk function from an Italian population study. *Eur Heart J* 2000; **21**: 365-370.

6: Pocock SJ, McCormack V, Gueyffier F, *et al*. A score for prediction risk from cardiovascular disease in adults with raised blood pressure, based upon individual patient data from random controlled trials. *Br Med J* 2001; **323**: 75-81.

7: Grover SA, Paquet S, Levington C, *et al*. Estimating the benefits of modifying risk factors of cardiovascular disease: a comparison of primary vs. secondary prevention. *Arch Intern Med* 1998; **158**: 655-662.

8: Conroy RM, Pyorala K, Fitzgerald AP, *et al*. for the SCORE project group. Estimation of ten-year risk of fatal cardiovascular disease in Europe: the SCORE Project. *Eur Heart J* 2003; **24**: 987-1003.

9: Turner RC, Millns H, Neil HAW, Stratton IM, Manley SE, Matthews DR, *et al.* Risk factors for coronary artery disease in non-insulin dependent diabetes mellitus. United Kingdom Prospective Diabetes Study (UKPDS 23). *Br Med J* 1998; **316**: 823-828.

10: Stevens RJ, Kothari V, Adler AI, Stratton IM, Holman RR on behalf of the United Kingdom Prospective Diabetes Study (UKPDS) Group. The UKPDS risk engine: a model for the risk of coronary heart disease in Type II diabetes (UKPDS 56). *Clin Sci* 2001; **101**: 671-679.

11: Despres J-P, Lemieur I, Prud'homme D. Treatment of obesity: need to focus on high risk abdominally obese patients. *Br Med J* 2001; **322**: 716-720.

12: Connor H, Annan F, Bunn E, *et al* for the Nutritional Subcommittee of the Diabetes Care Advisory Committee of Diabetes UK. The implementation of nutritional advice for people with diabetes. *Diab Med* 2003; **20**: 786-807.

13: O'Brien E, Beevers G, Lip GYH. ABC of hypertension. Blood pressure measurement. Part IV. Automated sphygmomanmetry: self blood pressure measurement. *Br Med J* 2001; **322**: 1167-1170 (12 May).

14: O'Brien E, Asmar R, Beilin L, *et al.* European Society of Hypertension Working Group on Blood Pressure Monitoring. European Society of Hypertension recommendations for conventional, ambulatory and home blood pressure measurement. *J Hypertension* 2003; **21**:821-848.

15: Fuller guidelines are available online: www.bhsoc.org

16: Rohlfing CL, Wiedmeyer HM, Little RR, *et al.* Defining the relationship between plasma glucose and HbA1c: analysis of glucose profiles and HbA1c in the Diabetes Control and Complications Trial. *Diab Care* 2002; **25**: 275-278.

17: Lawton J, Peel E, Douglas M, Parry O. "Urine testing is a waste of time": newly diagnosed type 2 diabetes patients' perceptions of self-monitoring. *Diab Med* 2004; **21**: 1045-1048.

18: Reynolds RM, Strachan MWJ. Editorial: Home blood glucose monitoring in type 2 diabetes. *Br Med J* 2004; **329**: 754-755 (2 October).

19: Russell M, Martier, SS, Sokol, RJ, *et al.* Screening for pregnancy risk drinking: TWEAKING the tests. *Alcoholism Clin Exp Res* 1991; **15(2)**: 638.

20: Chan, AWK, Pristach, EA, Welte JW, Russell M. Use of the TWEAK test in screening for alcoholism/heavy drinking in three populations. *Alcoholism Clin Exp Res* 1993; **17(6)**: 1188-1192.

21: Marshall SM. Screening for microalbuminuria: which measurement? *Diab Med* 1991; **8(8)**: 706-11.

22: Levene LS, McNally PG, Fraser RC, Lowy AGJ. What characteristics are associated with screening positive for microalbuminuria in patients with diabetes in the community? *Pract Diab Internat* 2004; **21**: 287-292.

Chapter 4 references

1: General Practice Committee. The New GP Contract. GPC 2003.

2: American Diabetes Association: Position Statement. Standards of Medical Care in Diabetes. *Diab Care* 2005; **28 (Supplement 1)**: S4-S36.

3: Ruderman N, Devlin JT, Schneider SH (editors). *Handbook of Exercise in Diabetes, 2nd Edition*. Alexandria, VA: American Diabetes Association 2002.

4: Department of Health. At Least Five a Week: evidence on the impact of physical activity and its relationship to health. A report from the Chief Medical Officer. London: HMSO, 2004.

5: North of England Hypertension Guideline Development Group. *Evidence-based Clinical Practice Guideline: Essential hypertension: managing adults in primary care*. London: HMSO National Institute of Clinical Excellence, August 2004.

6: Scottish Intercollegiate Guidelines Network. Management of Diabetes: A national clinical guideline (55). Edinburgh: Royal College of Physicians, 2001. Online. Available: http:www.sign.ac.uk

7: Hutchinson A, McIntosh A, Griffiths CJ, *et al*. Clinical guidelines and evidence review for Type 2 diabetes. Blood pressure management. Sheffield: ScHARR, University of Sheffield, 2002. Online. Available: http://shef.ac.uk/guidelines

8: Adler AI, Stratton IM, Neil HAW, *et al*. Association of systolic blood pressure with macrovascular and microvascular complications of type 2 diabetes (UKPDS 36): prospective observational study. *Br Med J* 2000; **321**: 412-419.

9: Williams B, Poulter NR, Brown MJ, *et al*. Guidelines for management of hypertension: report of the fourth working party of the British Hypertension Society, 2004- BHS IV. *J Hum Hypertension* 2004; **18**: 139-185.

10: McIntosh A, Hutchinson A, Feder G, *et al*. Clinical guidelines and evidence review for Type 2 diabetes. Lipids management. Sheffield: ScHARR, University of Sheffield, 2002. Online. Available: http://shef.ac.uk/guidelines

11: British Cardiac Society, British Hyperlipidaemia Association, British Hypertension Society, and endorsed by the British Diabetic Association. Joint British recommendations on prevention of coronary heart disease in clinical practice. *Heart* 1998; **80 (Supplement 2)**: S1-S29.

12: Collins R, Armitage J, Parish S, *et al* for the Heart Protection Study Collaborative Group. MRC / BHF Heart Protection Study of cholesterol lowering with simvastatin in 20 536 high-risk individuals: a randomised placebo-controlled trial. *Lancet* 2002; **360**:9326: 7-22 (6 July).

13: Colhoun HM, Betteridge DJ, Durrington PN, *et al*. Primary prevention of cardiovascular disease with atorvastatin in type 2 diabetes in the Collaborative Atorvastatin Diabetes Study (CARDS): a randomised placebo-controlled trial. *Lancet* 2004; **364**: 685-696.

14: McIntosh A, Hutcinson A, Home PD, *et al*. Clinical guidelines and evidence review for Type 2 diabetes: management of blood glucose. Sheffield: ScHARR, University of Sheffield, 2002. Online. Available: http://shef.ac.uk/guidelines

15: Winocour PH. Effective diabetes care: a need for realistic targets. *Br Med J* 2002; **324**: 1577-1580 (29 June).

16: Wright EC. Non-compliance – or how many aunts has Matilda?. *Lancet* 1993; **342**: 909-13.

17: Law MR, Wald NJ. Risk factor thresholds: their existence under scrutiny. *Br Med J* 2002; **324**: 1370-1376 (29 June).

Chapter 5 references

1: Wade DT, Halligan PW. Do biomedical models of illness make for good healthcare systems? *Br Med J* 2004; **329**: 1398-1401.

2: Gask L, Usherwood T. ABC of psychological medicine: The consultation. *Br Med J* 2002; **324**: 1567-1569 (29 June).

3: Pendleton D, Schofield T, Tate P *et al. The New Consultation: Developing Doctor-Patient Communication*. Oxford: Oxford University Press, 2003.

4: Launer J. *Narrative-based Primary Care: A Practical Guide*. Oxford: Radcliffe Medical Press, 2002.

5: Prochaska JO, DiClemente CC. Stages of change in the modification of problem behaviors. *Prog Behav Mod*. 1992; **28**: 183-218.

6: Richardson P. Psychological treatments. In: Davies T, Craig TKJ (Ed.). *ABC of Mental Health*. London: BMJ Books, 1998.

7: American Diabetes Association: Position Statement. Standards of Medical Care in Diabetes. *Diab Care* 2005; **28 (Supplement 1)**: S4-S36.

8: Lancaster T, Stead L, Silagy C, *et al* for the Cochrane Tobacco Addiction Review Group. Regular review: Effectiveness of interventions to help people stop smoking: findings from Cochrane. *Br Med J* 2000 (5 August); **321**: 355-358.

9: NICE Appraisal Committee. Technology Appraisal Guidance No. 39: Guidance on the use of nicotine replacement therapy (NRT) and bupropion for smoking cessation. London: NHS National Institute for Clinical Excellence March 2002. Online. Available: http://www.nice.org.uk

10: Online. Available: www.dh.gov.uk/PolicyAndGuidance/HealthAndSocialCareTopics/Tobacco/fs/en

11: Online. Available: www.givingupsmoking.co.uk

12: The University of York-NHS Centre for Reviews and Dissemination. Smoking cessation: What the health service can do. *Effectiveness Matters* 1998: **3** (1).

13: Silagy C, Mant D, Fowler G, *et al*. Nicotine replacement therapy for smoking cessation. In: Cochrane Library. Oxford: Update Software, 1998; issue 2. Updated quarterly.

14: Connor H, Annan F, Bunn E, *et al* for the Nutritional Subcommittee of the Diabetes Care Advisory Committee of Diabetes UK. The implementation of nutritional advice for people with diabetes. *Diabetic Medicine* 2003; **20**: 786-807.

15: Sacks FM, *et al*. Effects on blood pressure of reduced dietary sodium and the Dietary Approaches to Stop Hypertension (DASH) diet. DASH-Sodium Collaborative Research Group. *N Engl J of Medicine* 2001; **344**: 3-10.

16: Online. Available: http://www.nhlbi.nih.gov/health/public/heart/hbp/dash.

17: DAFNE Study Group. Training in flexible, intensive insulin management to enable dietary freedom in people with type 1 diabetes: dose adjustment for normal eating (DAFNE) randomised controlled trial. *Br Med J* 2002; **325**: 746-749.

18: American Diabetes Association Position Statement: Physical Activity/Exercise and Diabetes. *Diab Care* 2004; **27 (Supplement 1)**: S58-S62.

19: American Diabetes Association: Diabetes and exercise: the risk-benefit profile. In: *The Health Professional's Guide to Diabetes and Exercise*. Devlin JT, Ruderman N, (eds). Alexandria, VA, American Diabetes Association, 1995, p. 3–4.

20: NICE Appraisal Committee. Technology Appraisal Guidance No. 22: Guidance on the use of orlistat for the treatment of obesity in adults. London: NHS National Institute for Clinical Excellence March 2001. Online. Available: www.nice.org.uk

21: NICE Appraisal Committee. Technology Appraisal Guidance No. 31: Guidance on the use of sibutramine for the treatment of obesity in adults. London: NHS National Institute for Clinical Excellence October 2001. Online. Available: www.nice.org.uk

22: Data presented to American Heart Association Scientific Sessions November 2004.

23: Campbell L, Rössner S. Management of obesity in patients with type 2 diabetes. Diab Med 2001; 18: 345-354.

24: Sjöström L, Lindroos A-K, Peltonen M, *et al.* Lifestyle, Diabetes, and Cardiovascular Risk Factors 10 Years after Bariatric Surgery. *N Engl J Med* 2004; **351**: 2683-2693.

25: Williams B, Poulter NR, Brown MJ, *et al.* Guidelines for management of hypertension: report of the fourth working party of the British Hypertension Society, 2004. BHS IV. *J Hum Hypertension* 2004; **18**: 139-185.

26: North of England Hypertension Guideline Development Group. Evidence-based Clinical Practice Guideline: Essential hypertension: managing adults in primary care. London: HMSO National Institute of Clinical Excellence, August 2004.

27: Luft FC. Mechanisms and cardiovascular damage in hypertension. *Hypertension* 2001; **37**: 594-598.

28: Carlberg B, Samuelsson O, Lindholm LH. Atenolol in hypertension: is it a wise choice? *Lancet* 2004; **364**: 1684-1689.

29: Estacio RO, Jeffers BW, Hiatt WR, *et al.* The effect of nisoldipine as compared with enalapril on cardiovascular events in patients with non-insulin-dependent diabetes and hypertension. *N Engl J Med* 1998; **338**: 645-652.

30: Ramsay LE, Williams B, Johnston GD, *et al.* British Hypertension Society guidelines for hypertension management 1999: summary. *Br Med J* 1999; **319**: 630-635 (4 September).

31: Hutchinson A, McIntosh A, Griffiths CJ, *et al.* Clinical guidelines and evidence review for Type 2 diabetes. Blood pressure management. Sheffield: ScHARR, University of Sheffield, 2002. Online. Available: http://shef.ac.uk/guidelines

32: Hood S, *et al.* High prevalence of aldosterone-sensitive hypertension in unselected patients. *Q J Medicine* 2002; **95**: 621.

33: Tatti P, Pahor M, Byington PB, *et al.* Outcome results of the Fosinopril Versus Amlodipine Cardiovascular Events Randomized Trial (FACET) in patients with hypertension and NIDDM. *Diab Care* 1998; **21**: 597-603.

34: Pepine CJ, Handberg EM, Cooper-De-Hoff RM, *et al.* A calcium antagonist vs. a non-calcium antagonist hypertension treatment strategy for patients with coronary artery disease: the International Verapamil-Trandolapril Study (INVEST): a randomized controlled trial. *J Am Med* Assoc 2003; **290**: 2805-2816.

35: Heart Outcomes Prevention Evaluation Study Investigators. Effects of ramipril on cardiovascular and microvascular outcomes in patients with diabetes mellitus: results of the HOPE study and the MICRO-HOPE study. *Lancet* 2000; **355**: 253-259.

36: PROGRESS group: Randomised trial of a perindopril-based blood-pressure-lowering regimen among 6,105 individuals with previous stroke or transient ischaemic attack. *Lancet* 2001; **358**: 1033-1041.

37: Lindholm LH, Ibsen H, Dahlof B, *et al.* Cardiovascular morbidity and mortality in patients with diabetes in the Losartan Intervention For Endpoint reduction in hypertension study (LIFE): a randomised trial against atenolol. *Lancet* 2002; **359**: 1004-1010.

38: University of York Centre for Reviews and Dissemination. Effective Health Care: Effectiveness of antihypertensive drugs in black people. **8 (4)**, 2004. Online. Available: http://www.york.ac.uk/inst/crd/ehc84.pdf

39: ALLHAT Collaborative Research Group. Major cardiovascular events in hypertensive patients randomized to doxazosin vs chlorthalidone: the antihypertensive and lipid-lowering treatment to prevent heart attack trial (ALLHAT). *J Am Med Assoc* 2000; **283**: 1967-1975.

40: UK Prospective Diabetes Study Group. Efficacy of atenolol and captopril in reducing risk of macro vascular and micro vascular complications in type 2 diabetes: UKPDS 39. *Br Med J* 1998; **317**: 713-720.

41: ALLHAT Collaborative Research Group. Major outcomes in high-risk hypertensive patients randomized to angiotensin-converting enzyme inhibitor or calcium channel blocker vs. diuretic: The Antihypertensive and Lipid-Lowering Treatment to Prevent Heart Attacks Trial. *J Am Med* Assoc 2002; **288**: 2981-2997.

42: Blood Pressure Lowering Treatment Trialists' Collaboration. Effects of different blood-pressure-lowering regimens on major cardiovascular events: results of prospectively designed overviews of randomised trials. *Lancet* 2003; **362**: 1527-1545.

43: Dahöf B, Server PS, Poulter NR, *et al* for the ASCOT Investigators. Prevention of cardiovascular events with an antihypertensive regimen of amlodipine adding perindopril as required, in the Anglo-Scandinavian Cardiac Outcomes Trial-Blood Pressure Lowering Arm (ASCOT-BPLA): a multicentre randomised controlled trial. *Lancet* 2005; **366**: 895-906.

44: McIntosh A, Hutchinson A, Feder G, *et al.* Clinical guidelines and evidence review for Type 2 diabetes. Lipids management. Sheffield: ScHARR, University of Sheffield, 2002. Online. Available: http://shef.ac.uk/guidelines

45: Report from the Committee of Principal Investigators. A cooperative trial in the primary prevention of ischaemic heart disease using clofibrate. *Br Heart J.* 1978;**40**:1069-1103.

46: Koskinen P, Manttair M, Manninen V, *et al.* Coronary heart disease incidence in NIDDM patients in the Helsinki Heart Study. *Diabetes Care.* 1992;**15**:820-825.

47: Heinonen OP, Huttunen JK, Manninen V, *et al.* The Helsinki Heart Study: coronary heart disease incidence during an extended follow-up. *J Intern Med.* 1994; **235**: 41-49.

48: Rubins HB, Robins SJ, Collins D, *et al.* Gemfibrozil for the secondary prevention of coronary heart disease in men with low levels of high-density lipoprotein cholesterol: Veterans Affairs High-Density Lipoprotein Cholesterol Intervention Trial Study Group. *N Engl J Med.* 1999; **341**: 410-418.

49: The FIELD Study Investigators. The need for a large-scale trial of fibrate therapy in diabetes: the rationale and design of the Fenofibrate Intervention and Event Lowering in Diabetes (FIELD) study. *Cardiovascular Diabetology* 2004; **3**: 9.

50: Heart Protection Study Collaborative Group: MRC/BHF Heart Protection Study of cholesterol-lowering with simvastatin in 5963 people with diabetes: a randomised placebo-controlled trial. *Lancet* 2003: **361**: 2005-2016.

51: Colhoun HM, Betteridge DJ, Durrington PN, *et al.* Primary prevention of cardiovascular disease with atorvastatin in type 2 diabetes in the Collaborative Atorvastatin Diabetes Study (CARDS): a randomised placebo-controlled trial. *Lancet* 2004; **364**: 685-696.

52: Sever PS, Dahlof B, Poulter NR, *et al*; ASCOT investigators. Prevention of coronary and stroke events with atorvastatin in hypertensive patients who have average or lower-than- average cholesterol concentrations, in the Anglo-Scandanavian Cardiac Outcomes Trial--Lipid Lowering Arm (ASCOT-LLA): a multicentre randomised controlled trial. *Lancet* 2003; **361**: 1149-1158.

53: Ezetimibe - a new cholesterol-lowering drug. *Drug Thera Bull*, September 2004; **42(9)**: 65-67.

54: American Diabetes Association Position Statement: Dyslipidemia Management in Adults with Diabetes. *Diab Care* 2004; **27 (Supplement 1)**: S68-S71.

55: Winocour PH, Fisher M. Prediction of cardiovascular risk in people with diabetes. *Diab Med* 2003; **20**: 515-527.

56: Levene LS. *Management of Type 2 Diabetes Mellitus in Primary Care*: A Practical Guide. Edinburgh: Butterworth Heinemann, 2003.

57: NICE Guideline Development Group and Recommendations Panel. Inherited Clinical Guideline G. Management of type 2 diabetes: Management of blood glucose. London: NHS National Institute for Clinical Excellence September 2002. Online. Available: http://www.nice.org.uk

58: UKPDS Study Group: U.K. Prospective Diabetes Study 16. Overview of 6 years' therapy of type II diabetes: a progressive disease. *Diabetes* 1995; **44**: 1249-58

59: UK Prospective Diabetes Study (UKPDS) Group. Intensive blood-glucose control with sulphonylureas or insulin compared with conventional treatment and risk of complications in patients with type II diabetes (UKPDS 33). *Lancet* 1998; **352**: 837-853.

60: Krentz AJ, Bailey CJ, Melander A. Thiazolidinediones for type 2 diabetes (Editorial). *Br Med J* 2000 (29 July); **321**: 252-253.

61: Day C. Thiazolidinediones: a new class of antidiabetic drugs. *Diab Med* 1999; **16**: 179-192.

62: NICE Appraisal Committee. Technology Appraisal Guidance No. 63: Guidance on the use of glitazones for the treatment of type 2 diabetes. London: NHS National Institute for Clinical Excellence August 2003. Online. Available: http://www.nice.org.uk

63: Bailey CJ, Day C, Krentz A. Nice timing for glitazones. *Br J Diab Vasc Dis* 2003; **3**: 308-309.

64: Higgs ER, Kretz AJ on behalf of the Association of British Clinical Diabetologists. ABCD position statement on glitazones. *Pract Diab Internat* 2004; **27**: 293–295.

65: Goldberg RB, *et al.* A comparison of glycemic effects of pioglitazone and rosiglitazone in patients with Type 2 diabetes and dyslipidemia. American Heart Association Scientific Session November 2004.

66: Skyler, JS. Effects of Glycemic Control on Diabetes Complications and on Prevention of Diabetes. *Clinical Diabetes* 2004; **22**: 162-166

67: Krentz A J, Bailey C J. *Type 2 Diabetes in Practice*. London: Royal Society of Medicine Press Limited 2001.

68: American Diabetes Association Clinical Practice Recommendations. Position Statement: Insulin Administration. *Diab Care* 2000; **23 (Supplement 1)**: S86-89.

69 American Diabetes Association Position Statement: Aspirin Therapy in Diabetes. *Diab Care* 2004; **27 (Supplement 1)**: S72-S73.

70: CAPRIE Steering Committee. A randomized, blinded trial of clopidogrel versus aspirin in patients at risk of ischemic events (CAPRIE). *Lancet* 1996; **348**: 1329-1339.

71: Diabetes UK Care recommendation: Aspirin treatment in Diabetes. Available: http://www.diabetes.org.uk/infocentre/carerec/aspirin.htm

72: Parving H-H, Hommel E, Smidt UM. Protection of kidney function and decrease in albumin by captopril in insulin dependent diabetics with nephropathy. *Br Med J* 1988; **297**: 1086-91.

73: Bjork S, Mulec H, Johnsen SA, Norden G, Aurell M. Renal protective effect of enalapril in diabetic nephropathy. *Br Med J* 1992; **304**: 339-43.

74: Ravid M, Savin H, Jutrin I, Bental T, Katz B, Lishner M. Long-term stabililizing effect of Angiotensin-converting enzyme inhibition on Plasma creatinine and on Proteinuria in normotensive Type 2 diabetic patients. *Ann Int Med* 1993; **118(8)**: 557-581.

75: Brenner BM, Cooper ME, de Zeeuw D *et al.* Effects of losartan on renal and cardiovascular outcomes in patients with type 2 diabetes and nephropathy. *N Engl J Med* 2001; **345**: 861-869.

76: Chugh A, Eagle KA, Mehta RH. Cardiac Complications and Management In Williams R, Herman W, Kinmouth A-L, *et al*, editors. *The Evidence Base for Diabetes Care.* Chichester: John Wiley & Sons, Ltd, 2002.

Index